Otolaryngology Research Advances

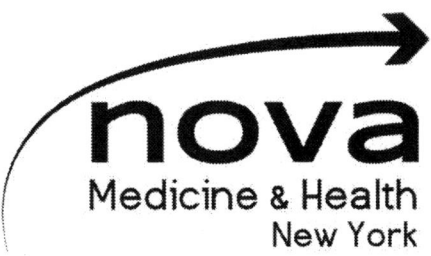

Otolaryngology Research Advances

Deafness: Current Perspectives and Research Developments
Sujeet Kumar Sinha, PhD (Editor)
Niraj Kumar Singh, PhD (Editor)
Animesh Barman, PhD (Editor)
2022. ISBN: 978-1-68507-980-2 (Hardcover)
2022. ISBN: 979-8-88697-075-3 (eBook)

Atlas of Salivary Glands Diseases
Salma Mohammed Al Sheibani, MD, Mohammed Jamil Hyder, MD and Subirendra Kumar, MD (Authors)
2021. ISBN: 978-1-68507-227-8 (Online Book)

Nasal and Paranasal Sinus Surgery: State of the Art and Future Perspectives
Francesco Gazia, MD (Editor)
Francesco Galletti, MD, PhD and Ordinary Professor (Editor)
Bruno Galletti, MD, PhD (Editor)
Francesco Freni, MD, PhD (Editor)
2021. ISBN: 978-1-53619-744-0 (Hardcover)
2021. ISBN: 978-1-53619-848-5 (eBook)

Salivary Glands: Structure, Functions and Regulation
Alicia S. Bryant (Editor)
2020. ISBN: 978-1-53617-497-7 (Softcover)
2020. ISBN: 978-1-53618-800-4 (eBook)

Ototoxicity: Signs, Symptoms and Treatment
Gregg Colon (Editor)
2019. ISBN: 978-1-53616-396-4 (Softcover)
2019. ISBN: 978-1-53616-417-6 (eBook)

More information about this series can be found at
https://novapublishers.com/product-category/series/otolaryngology-research-advances/

Anisha Webb
Editor

Maxillary Sinus Diseases

From Diagnosis to Treatment

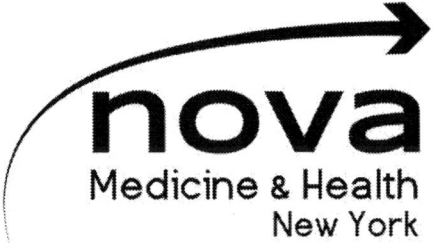

Copyright © 2024 by Nova Science Publishers, Inc.

All rights reserved. No part of this book may be reproduced, stored in a retrieval system or transmitted in any form or by any means: electronic, electrostatic, magnetic, tape, mechanical photocopying, recording or otherwise without the written permission of the Publisher.

We have partnered with Copyright Clearance Center to make it easy for you to obtain permissions to reuse content from this publication. Please visit copyright.com and search by Title, ISBN, or ISSN.

For further questions about using the service on copyright.com, please contact:

Copyright Clearance Center
Phone: +1-(978) 750-8400   Fax: +1-(978) 750-4470   E-mail: info@copyright.com

NOTICE TO THE READER

The Publisher has taken reasonable care in the preparation of this book but makes no expressed or implied warranty of any kind and assumes no responsibility for any errors or omissions. No liability is assumed for incidental or consequential damages in connection with or arising out of information contained in this book. The Publisher shall not be liable for any special, consequential, or exemplary damages resulting, in whole or in part, from the readers' use of, or reliance upon, this material. Any parts of this book based on government reports are so indicated and copyright is claimed for those parts to the extent applicable to compilations of such works.

Independent verification should be sought for any data, advice or recommendations contained in this book. In addition, no responsibility is assumed by the Publisher for any injury and/or damage to persons or property arising from any methods, products, instructions, ideas or otherwise contained in this publication.

This publication is designed to provide accurate and authoritative information with regards to the subject matter covered herein. It is sold with the clear understanding that the Publisher is not engaged in rendering legal or any other professional services. If legal or any other expert assistance is required, the services of a competent person should be sought. FROM A DECLARATION OF PARTICIPANTS JOINTLY ADOPTED BY A COMMITTEE OF THE AMERICAN BAR ASSOCIATION AND A COMMITTEE OF PUBLISHERS.

Library of Congress Cataloging-in-Publication Data

ISBN: 979-8-89113-534-5

Published by Nova Science Publishers, Inc. † New York

Contents

Preface		vii
Chapter 1	**The Rare and Uncommon Pathology of Maxillary Sinus**	1
	Smail Kharoubi	
Chapter 2	**Odontogenic-Related Maxillary Sinusitis: Unraveling Microbial Dynamics and Preventive Strategies in Multidisciplinary Care**	45
	Hema Suryawanshi and Santosh R. Patil	
Chapter 3	**The Role of Maxillary Sinus in Dental Infections: A Review of Current Knowledge and Clinical Implications**	63
	Santosh R. Patil and Mohmed Isaqali Karobari	
Chapter 4	**Maxillary Sinus Hypoplasia**	79
	Mohammad Hatamleh, Zain Al-Qudah, Mohammad Khraisat, Ra'ed Al-ashqar and Mohannad Al-Qudah	
Chapter 5	**Maxillary Sinusitis of Dental Origin**	93
	Mosaad Abdel-Aziz and Ayman S. Megahed	
Index		107

Preface

This book consists of five chapters that explore the diagnosis to treatment of maxillary sinus diseases. The aim of Chapter One is to discuss some of these rare and uncommon pathologies of maxillary sinus and their management. Chapter Two serves as a comprehensive guide for clinicians, researchers, and dental healthcare providers involved in the multidisciplinary care of individuals at risk for odontogenic-related maxillary sinusitis. Chapter Three provides a comprehensive overview of maxillary sinusitis in the context of dental infections. The rare condition, maxillary sinus hypoplasia, is discussed in Chapter Four. The last chapter reviews maxillary sinusitis of dental origin.

Chapter 1

The Rare and Uncommon Pathology of Maxillary Sinus

Smail Kharoubi[*]

Department of ENT and Facial Surgery, Hospital Dr Dorban - Hospital University Center (Chu), Annaba, Algeria
Faculty of Medicine, University Badji Mokhtar, Annaba, Algeria

Abstract

The maxillary sinus is a bilateral paranasal cavity that enlarges until the age of 7 or 9, and is traversed by a respiratory mucosa with a small opening: the middle meatus.

The maxillary sinus can present many and various pathologies: congenital, infectious, traumatic, tumoral (benign or malignant), and iatrogenic.

Diagnosing of these pathologies requires a clinical exam with endoscopy, imaging (CT-scan, RMN), biologic investigation, and biopsy.

There are also many rare and uncommon pathologies, such as specific infections, autoimmune diseases and inflammatory fibrous tumors, which are recognized after difficult and complex management.

The aim of this chapter is to discuss some of these rare and uncommon pathologies of maxillary sinus and their management.

Keywords: maxillary sinus, auto immune disease, agenesis, sinus endoscopy, middle meatotomy, CT scan, foreign body maxillary sinus

---

[*] Corresponding Author's Email: smail.kharoubi17@gmail.com.

In: Maxillary Sinus Diseases
Editor: Anisha Webb
ISBN: 979-8-89113-534-5
© 2024 Nova Science Publishers, Inc.

1. Introduction

The maxillary sinus is an aerial cavity present from the age of 4 years (maxillary antrum) and annexed to the nasal fossa. The maxillary sinus is bilateral and symmetrical, and lined with respiratory mucosa and communicates with the nasal cavity through an orifice known as the middle meat. The maxillary sinus can be clinically examined from the anterior part (inspection, palpation) and from the inside part (nasal endoscopy). Examination of the cavity itself requires endoscopy via an inferior, middle meatotomy, or after bone trepanation via the vestibular approach.

Imaging is a fundamental element in the evaluation of the various medical and surgical pathologies of the maxillary sinuses. CT scans enable visualization of the cavity lumen, walls as well as the sinus environment. MRI refines the diagnosis of tissue lesions and the behavior of neighboring structures (endocranial orbits).

The pathology of the maxillary sinus is dominated by acute and chronic infections (viral, bacterial, and mycotic), followed by a wide variety of benign and malignant tumors (dominated by epithelial and vascular varieties), traumatology, medical and surgical iatrogenic.

The maxillary sinuses are also affected by rare or even exceptional conditions, either as revelations or during the course of a known, ongoing disease. The maxillary sinus may therefore represent a particular stage in the evolution of a regional or general diseases, and may sometimes require specialized expertise and adapted management to improve a medical outcome, avoid a complication, or even anticipate or attenuate the severity or aggressiveness of a disease.

This chapter therefore presents a necessarily exhaustive catalog or user manual for dealing with rare and unusual diseases of the maxillary sinuses.

2. Examination and Exploration of Maxillary Sinus

2.1. Physical Examination

- *Inspection:* It is the first staple. Practitioner inspect the face (anterior wall) and relate all modification like congestion, eruptive lesion, swelling, ulceration, mass, and the presence of exophthalmia or nasal anomalies especially nostril, upper lip and nasogenien furrow.

- *Palpation:* the aim is to search for a facial mass, painful, unclenched by palpation or osteolysis. Nerve testing: the neurologic exam tested especially the trigeminal nerve V1 V2 V3 and research anesthesia or hypoesthesia.
- *Oral cavity exam*: the examination of the oral cavity offered an access to the inferior face of the maxillary sinus. We research a palatal modification (swelling, perforation, ulceration).

2.2. Objective Investigation

- Nasal endoscopy authorizes evaluation of endonasal cavity, the right and left side of septum in anterior, medium and posterior parts. We can appreciate architectural, mucous and neoformations. In this procedure, we make different sampling; bacteriology, cytology (eosinophilic cell), or biopsy if necessary.
- *Sinus endoscopy*: After inferior meatus by contact anesthesia (naphtazolin xylocain 5%) and mucous infiltrating (adrenalin xylocain). We introduce endoscopal sinus after inferior meatotomy and notified aspect of intra sinusal mucous, cysts, tumor, secretions, fungal lesion and make all sampling (bacteriology, cytology) or endosinusal biopsy.

2.3. Imaging

- Ultrasonography (A-Mode): (Figure 1) [1]

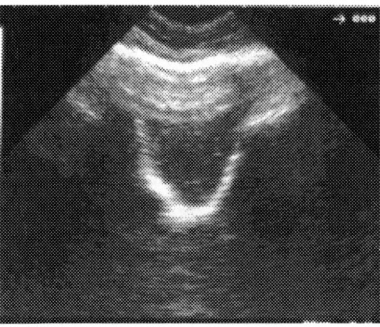

Figure 1. Maxillary sinus Ultrasonography (normal aspect).

- CT scan: (Figure 2, 3)

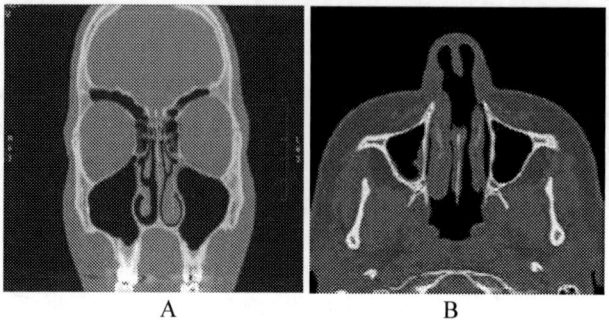

Figure 2. CT scan - Face. A: Coronal CT scan. Normal maxillary sinus. B: Axial CT scan. normal aspect of maxillary sinus.

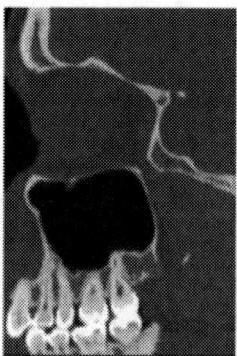

Figure 3. Sagittal CT scan. Normal aspect of maxillary sinus.

- MRI: (Figure 4)

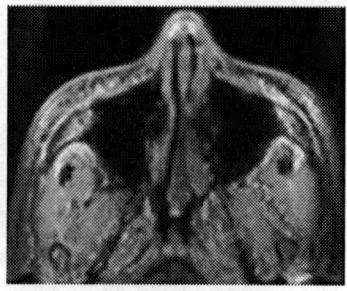

Figure 4. MRI axial view (normal maxillary sinus).

- Cone-Beam: (Figure 5, 6)

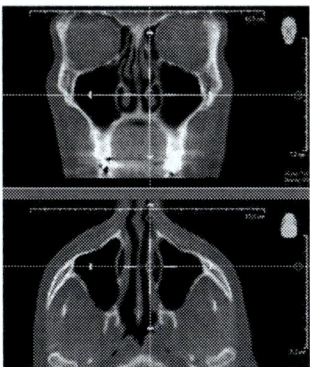

Figure 5. Cone-Beam nasosinusal cavities (normal maxillary sinus).

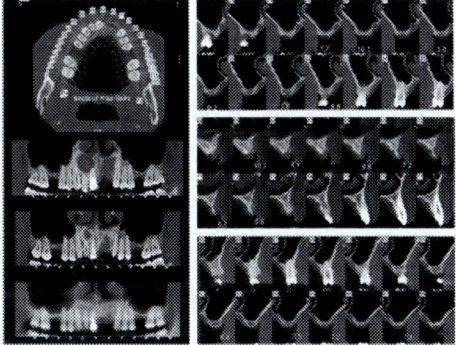

Figure 6. Cone-Beam sinuso dental incidence.

- 18FDG PET: (Figure 7)

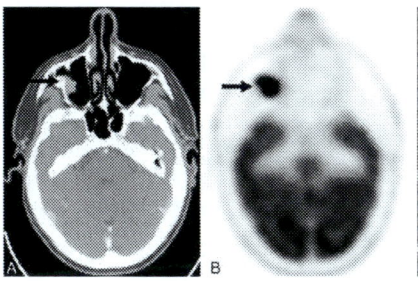

Figure 7. 18 FDG PET Face: maxillary benign tumor right maxillary sinus. Left maxillary sinus is normal.

3. Signs and Symptoms of Maxillary Sinus Diseases

Symptoms of maxillary sinus symptoms are not specific and common to all rhinologic disturbance. Nasal obstruction, rhinorrhea, epistaxis, facial pains, hyposmia or anosmia, nasal crusting, face swelling, palatal deformities, proptosis, dacryocystis, snoring, orofacial or palatal fistula (Table 1, 2).

Table 1. Symptoms and signs of maxillary sinus pathology

SINUSAL SYNDROME: nasal obstruction, rhinorrhea, epistaxis, hyposmia, anosmia.
ORBITAL SYNDROME: proptosis, diplopia.
BUCCAL SYNDROME: trismus, palatal perforation, palatal mass.
NEUROLOGIC SYNDROME: neurologic deficit (V), headache, facial pain, facial nevralgia.

Table 2. Maxillary sinus disease: Synthesis of different staple of management

1: MEDICAL HISTORY OF MAXILLARY SINUS DISEASE.
2: SIGNS AND SYMPTOMS OF DISEASE.
3: CLINICAL EXAM. INSPECTION, PALPATION ENDONASAL ENDOSCOPIC EXAM ORAL CAVITY EXAMINATION NEUROLOGIC EXAMINATION (V)
▼
4: SYNTHESIS OF THE CASE. INFECTIOUS SYNDROME / INFLAMMATORY SYNDROME/TUMORAL SYNDROME
▼
5: EXPLORATIONS.
▼
BIOLOGY ━━━━ IMAGING ━━━━ BIOPSY Ultrasounds-CT scan-MRI-18FGD PET.
▼
6: FINAL DIAGNOSIS AND TREATMENT OPTIONS.

Sometime the disease is recognize after screening complications; neurologic complications (meningitis, cerebral abscess, thrombophlebitis), orbitary complications (celullitis, sub periostal abscess, orbital abscess). Skin modifications (congestion or readless, ulceration, nodosity, induration, infiltration) is possible and inaugural cervical adenopathy is rare.

In another cases the discovery of maxillary sinus pathology is make fortunately after cheek imaging, dental radiography, bucco dental surgery or nasosinusal functional surgery.

4. Pathology

4.1. Congenital Anomalies of Maxillary Sinus

4.1.1. Agenesis of Maxillary Sinus

Maxillary sinus aplasia is a very rare congenital anomaly.

4.1.1.1. Aetiology
Agenesis of the maxillary sinus is a congenital anomaly caused by the absence of development of maxillary sinus (isolated or associated with other sinus).

4.1.1.2. Diagnosis
Agenesis of the maxillary sinus can occur esthetic defects in the face. Patients also report pain. In many cases the diagnosis is occurred by radiologic exam (Figure 8, 9).

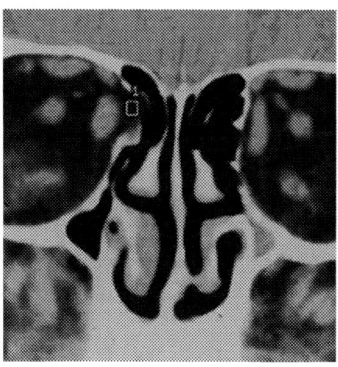

Figure 8. CT scan coronal view. Agenesis of left maxillary sinus.

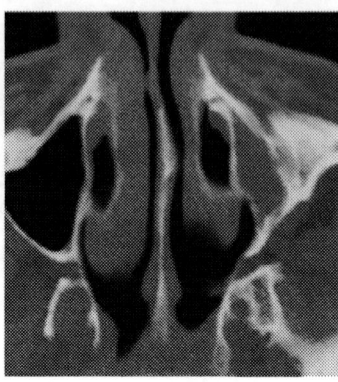

Figure 9. CT scan axial view. Agenesis of left maxillary sinus.

4.1.1.3. Evolution

Maxillary sinus agenesis is a non-evolving clinical and radiological finding that deserves to be identified so as not to be mistaken for pathology (sinusitis, tumor).

4.2. Hypoplasia Maxillary Sinus

Maxillary sinus hypoplasia is uncommon condition that may be misdiagnosed as chronic sinusitis with prevalence to be 1% -11%.

4.2.1. Aetiology

Hypoplasia in embryologic developpement: associated with some congenital anomalies (Apert, Crouzon, Treacher-Collins).

Hypoplasia acquired after traumatic, iatrogenic (surgery of maxillary sinus) or structural dysfunction.

4.2.2. Diagnosis

The hypoplasic maxillary sinus is discovered generally after recurrent sinusitis, post surgical pain, traumatic injury, or radiologic examination. Endonasal endoscopy is normal.

CT scan shows a consequent reduction of maxillary sinus volume without bone lysis (Figure 10).

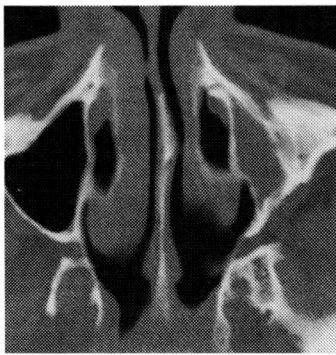

Figure 10. CT scan axial view. Hypoplasia of right maxillary sinus (agenesis of left maxillary).

4.2.3. Evolution

Maxillary sinus hypoplasia predisposes to lamina papyracea injuries and orbital penetration during endoscopic sinus surgery and dental problems (canine fossea elevation). It may clinically lead to silent sinus, ophtalmology disturbance (orbital asymmetry and double vision).

4.3. Maxillary Pneumosinus Dilatans

Pneumosinus dilatans is a rare condition resulting to abnormal enlargement of one or more paranasal sinuses. Pneumosinus dilatans can affect maxillary sinus in 20% of cases (1).

Maxillary sinus pneumocele was first described by Noyek in 1974 [2].

4.3.1. Aetiology

- congenital malformation.
- presence of spontaneously draining mucocele.
- dilatation by gas-forming microorganism.
- presence of one-way valve.

4.3.2. Diagnosis

Maxillary pneumosinus dilatans may be asymptomatic but cause a variety of symptoms (Table 3). The symptoms can be aggrieved after high altitude, nose blowing and sun exposure.

- Cosmetic complaint.
- Facial pain or pressure.
- Orbital displacement or proptosis.
- Nasal obstruction (displacement of neighboring structures).
- Others: otalgia, hearing loss, sneezing.

Table 3. Symptoms (classified by frequency) of maxillary pneumosinus dilatans

swelling
Proptosis
Facial pain
Nasal obstruction
Numbness
Visual problems
Asymptomatic
Toothache
Headache
Sinusitis

Furthermore pneumosinus dilatans of maxillary sinus is potentially (56%) associated to visions loss, arachnoid cysts (8%) and orbital tumor (4%) []).

In nasal endoscopy mucosa was normal without secretion.

CT scan showed hyper pneumatization of maxillary sinus, massive dilatation, medial displacement of membranous medial maxillary wall, superior displacement of orbital floor and thinning of zygomatic bone [3] (Figure 11).

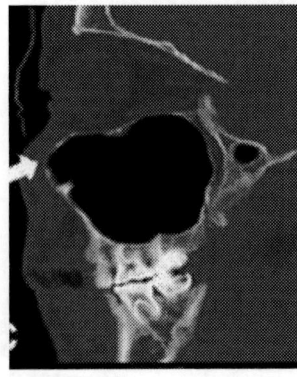

Figure 11. CT scan sagittal plan. Hyperpneumatization of maxillary sinus (with arrow).

Magnetic resonance imaging (MRI) exclude other differential diagnoses or associated pathology. 18F-NaF PET-CT scan helped in cases where the diagnosis is difficult (significant uptake by the walls affected by pneumosinus dilatans) [4].

4.3.3. Therapy

Treatment of maxillary pneumosinus dilatans consists of creation of a naso-antral window endoscopically or by Caldwell luc operation. Some authors choose a reconstruction of the anterior wall with titanium mesh and mini screw [5]. Hyun obtain good result after reduction osteoplasty [6]. Choi proposed electrical burring [7].

4.2.4. Evolution

Without treatment pneumosinus dilatans continued to developing and induce ophthalmologic and cosmetic complications.

5. Specific Infection

5.1. Tuberculosis of Maxillary Sinus

Tuberculosis is one of chronic diseases caused by a specific bacteria, mycobacterium tuberculosis and pulmonary localization is the most common presentation especially in third world countries or patients with deficit immunity status. The first case report is by Morgani in 1761 [8]. It is more frequent in females.

Nodes are the most site of extra pulmonary localization (15% of all sites). Tuberculosis of the paranasal sinus is rare in occurrence. The incidence of sinusal cases is low and forty cases as reported until 1977 [8].

5.1.1 Aetiology

Most cases of tubercular involvement of the maxillary sinus are secondary to pulmonary tuberculosis.

We recognize two ways from maxillary sinus inoculation:

- Direct or primitive form: Inoculation of tuberculosis involving the maxillary sinus usually
- Occurs directly (primitive form) though infected microdroplets.

- Indirect or secondary form: microbacterium occurs by another site (pulmonary, lymphatic).

5.1.2. Pathology

Pathologically, three phases can be recognized: first phase infection is confined to the mucousa (thickness, polyp, secretion). Second phase bony involvement and fistula formation and third phase with hyperplastic lesion and formation of tuberculoma.

5.1.3. Diagnosis

Symptoms are not specific and patients report nasal obstruction, rhinorrhea, nasal bleeding, deteriorated sense of smell and pain. Nocturne fever, night sweats, asthenia, anorexia, caught, facial swelling, can be noted and represent general signs of tuberculosis imprinting. The diagnosis can be recognize after histopathological study of chirurgical specimen (polyps, sinus mucosa, mucosal biopsy).

In another cases the maxillary sinus tuberculosis can mimicked an odontogenic infection arising maxillary (second and third molars) [9, 10, 11].

Nasal endoscopy shows a thickness of nasal mucosa, secretions, middle meatal polyps. Sinusal endoscopy (maxillary sinus) noted hypertrophic mucosa with secretion or polyps.

Imaging (CT scan) is not specific and report total or partial opacity of maxillary sinus, hypertrophic mucosa (unilateral), bony hypertrophy. Calcification within sinuses can be indicative of sinonasal tuberculosis but imaging findings are mostly non specific (Figure 12).

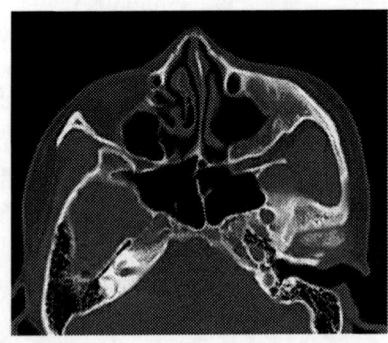

Figure 12. Axial paranasal CT scan: Tuberculous - mucoperiostal thickening in the left maxillary sinus.

Table 4. Diagnosis criteria of sinusitis tuberculous [9]

PARANASAL SINUS TUBERCULOSIS: CRITERIA.
- Absence of clinical response of empirical antibiotics. - Presence of caseous granulomatous inflammatory lesions on histopathology. - Identification of Mycobacterium tuberculosis in surgical specimen.

Table 5. Tuberculosis diagnosis

Tuberculin Skin Tests. Imaging (CT scan- MRN). Chest X-ray (pulmonary tuberculosis). Bacteriology direct exam: Ziehl Neelsen. Mycobacterium culturing. Polymerase Chain Reaction (PCR). Gene Xpert MTB/RIF. Histopathological examination (surgical specimen). Test treatment.

Diagnostic can be best made using a standard Mantoux test for tuberculosis, bacteriological study of secretions or maxillary mucous after direct exam (Zieel Nelsen) and especially growthly in specific area solid one like Lowenstein Jensen or liquid one like (Table 4).

Histopathological examination can reveal epithelioid and giant cells suggestive of tuberculosis but only the presence of caseation necrosis is pathognomonic (Figure 13) (Table 6).

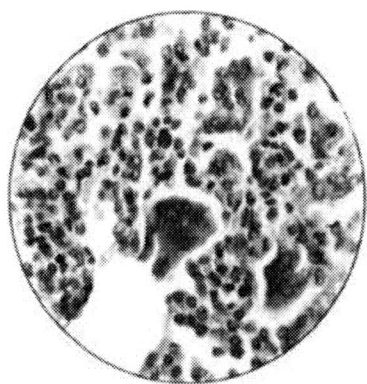

Figure 13. Histopathological pictures showing Langhan's cell.

Table 6. Differentially diagnosis in paranasal sinus tuberculosis

INFECTIOUS DISEASE:
   Syphilis
   Leprosy
   Actinomycosis. Coccidioidomycosis. Blastomycosis
   Leishmaniosis
NON INFECTIOUS DISEASE:
   Carcinoma. Lymphoma
   Wegener's granulomatosis
   Angiofibroma
   Sarcoidosis
   Periarteritis nodosa
   Castleman's disease
   Amyloidosis

5.1.4. Therapy

Treatment of tuberculosis is medical with antitubercular treatment regimes combining three or four drogues during six to nine months (Table 7).

Table 7. Treatment modalities of paranasal sinus tuberculosis

MEDICAL TREATMENT
Two (02) months:
   Isoniazid 5 mg/kg/j
   Rifampicin 10 mg/kg/j
   Pyrazinamide 30 mg/kg/j
   Ethambutol
Fourth (04) to Seven (07) months:
   Isoniazid
   Rifampicin
SURGICAL TREATMENT
Sinus drainage
Specimen collection
Complications
Sequels

Surgical treatment of tuberculosis of the maxillary sinus is an rarely choose in first line. It is recommended after poor medical treatment results, complications or sequels. Endonasal endoscopic way his habitually performed. In few cases external approach will be necessary (Caldwell-Luc operation, Degloving, Lateronasal procedure) [10, 12].

5.1.5. Evolution

Evolution after anti tubercular treatment is generally favorable. Without treatment the disease will be during and procure contagion, other localizations, osteolysis and decline of general health of patients.

5.2. Syphilis of Maxillary Sinus

Syhilis is infection caused by treponema pallidum and is classically divided into primary, secondary latent and tertiary stages.

5.2.1. Aetiology

Syphilis is caused by microbial agent, treponema pallidum and divided on two entities:

- Acquired syphilis (venereal disease): primary, secondary and early latent, late latent syphilis.
- Congenital syphilis.

5.2.2. Diagnosis

Primary syphilis: ulceration in nasal septum and adenopathy during few weeks.

Secondary syphilis: rhinorrhea, fever, headache. Endonasal exam shows red and ovoid plaques in anterior part of nasal septum and inferior turbinates.

Tertiary syphilis characterized by development of granulomatous lesions (syphilisis gomea). CT scan can identify bone lysis, especially in the roof of nasal cavities.

Biologic tests:

- Direct test of serous secretions: dark ground microscopy, PCR test: early syphilis.
- Serology of syphilis (Table 8).

Table 8. Lecture of results of the serology in syphilis disease

VRDL (-), TPHA (-) : absence of syphilis, precocity syphilis.
TPHA (-), VDRL (+) : others bacterial infections.
VRDL (-), TPHA (+) : syphilis cured, tertiary syphilis.
VRDL (+), TPAH (+) : active syphilis.

Quantitative tests: TPHA (treponema pallidum hemagglutination assay), FTA (fluorescent treponemal antibody).

Qualitative tests: VRDL (venereal disease research laboratory).

NB: FTA is the first positively test after primary infection followed by VRDL and finally TPHA tests.

5.2.3. Therapy

Antibiotherapy, penicillin class, is the gold standard for treatment of syphilis.

Primary, secondary, early latent syphilis:

- benzatine penicillin 2,4 megaunits (intramuscular single dose).
- procaine penicillin 600 00 units once day daily for 10 days.
- doxyxycline 100mg twice daily for 14 days.

Late latent syphilis:

- benzatine penicillin 2,4 megaunits (intramuscular, three injections over two weeks: days 0, 7, 14).
- procaine penicillin 900 00 units once day daily for 17 days.
- doxycycline 200mg twice daily for 28 days.

New treatment: azithromycin (2gr oral) is as effective treating early syphilis as benzatine penicillin.

5.2.4. Evolution

After acquire syphilis a significant risk of reinfection is possible and the regular serological screening is recommending.

Sequels can be seen and consist on nasal septum perforation, palatine perforation, destruction of osteo cartilaginous nasal structure, endonasal synechiae, crusting rhinitis.

5.3. Leprosy of Maxillary Sinus

Leprosy is a chronic infectious disease caused by Mycobacterium leprae that primarily affects the skin, the peripheral nerves, the upper respiratory tract, and the eyes.

5.3.1. Aetiology
Mycobacterium leprae is an acid-fast bacilli
    Nasal mucosal involvement is quite common in LL, likely because it is one of the main transmission sites for the bacillus.

5.3.2. Pathology:
The maxillary deformities in patients with leprosy are collectively termed facies leprosa or rhinomaxillary syndrome. The anterior nasal spine shows progressive resorption and resorption of the alveolar process leads the incisors, the palatine process shows bone erosion and perforation, and intranasal structures especially the turbinates and septum result in atrophy and perforation [13].

5.3.3. Diagnosis
The symptoms are not specific; nasal obstruction, rhinorrhea, epistaxis. Nasal endoscopy note mucosal congestion, muco-purulent secretions and limited decolorize mucous (head of middle turbinate). Nasal crusting is habitually associated with atrophic nasal structures.

    Imaging approach is necessary and a useful method for the evaluation of patient response to treatment and follow up. CT scan shows maxillary bone deformities and opacity of one or all sinus cavities. In fine the diagnosis of leprosy is based in skin exam (slit-skin smear, skin biopsy). PCR is also used to support the suspicion of diagnosis of leprosy a clinical [13].

5.3.4. Therapy
Multi- drug therapy is used associated rifanpicin-clofazimine-dapsone. We can utilize also ofloxacine, minocycline. Other chemotherapeutic agents: levofloxacin (LVFX), sparfloxacin (SPFX), and clarithromycin [14].

5.3.5. Evolution
Leprosy remains a serious infection that can leave serious functional and cosmetic effects, requiring following up, and verification (clinical, radiological, biological) of recovery.

6. Rare and Uncommun Tumor of Maxillary Sinus

6.1. Diagnosis Modalities of Maxillary Sinus Tumor

6.1.1. Clinical Semiology
The semiology of maxillary sinus tumors is nonspecific and reflects nasosinus dysfunction. Symptoms include nasal obstruction, rhinorrhea, epistaxis, facial pains and smell disorders. The palatal deformity may be seen also, and anterior jugal deformities (facial swelling).

Malignant variants may be further distinguished by persistent, severe pain, trismus, orbital manifestations (exophthalmos, oculo-motors paralysis), neurological deficits (Trigeminal nerve -V), intractable headache, and rarely revelatory cervical adenopathy or distant metastasis.

The persistence of any rhinosinual symptoms and its relapsing after treatment, together with the unilateral and progressive nature of the symptoms (involvement of neighboring structures), should draw attention to a nasosinusal tumor process.

6.1.2. Nasal Endoscopy
Endonasal endoscopic examination is the best procedure in the diagnosis (visualization) and evaluation of an endonasal tumor. After local anesthesia and retraction of the nasal cavity (naphthazoline xylocain 5%), a rigid 0° endoscop is used to visualize the tumor, its location, form and extensions. It can also be used for guided biopsies.

6.1.3. Imaging
Imaging is a fundamental complement in the diagnosis, treatment and follow-up of endonasal tumors (benign and malignant). It is based on a combination of CT and MRI scans. CT scans (axial, coronal and sagittal incidences) are used to diagnose the tumor, its boundaries, location and extensions (cerebral, infra-temporal fossa, orbits, oral cavity and anterior); tumor structure (homogeneous or heterogeneous) and vascular nature are analyzed after injection of contrast medium. MRI is used to refine tissue analysis, precise extensions and precise relationships with the orbit and cerebral neurovascular structures (Figure 14, 15).

Imaging is the better program in the surveillance of sinus tumors (especially malignant ones), and helps to recurrences identification.

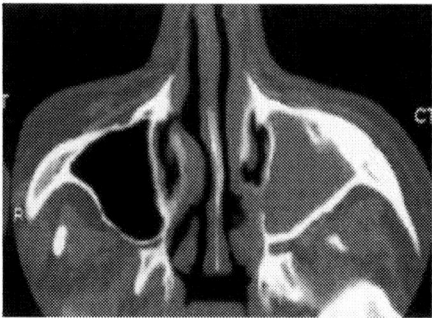

Figure 14. Axial CT scan: Respiratory epithelial adenomatoid hamartoma (REHA). (Iconography Di Carlo.R Ref [16]).

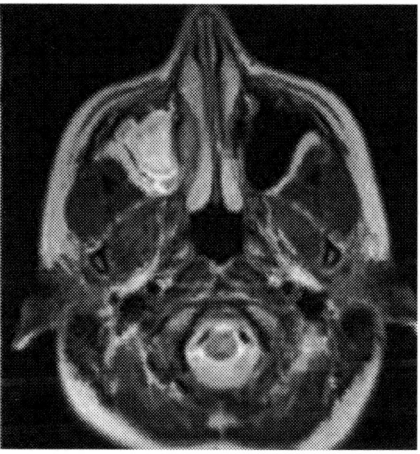

Figure 15. Axial MRI: Esthesioneuroblastoma Contrast enhancing lesion in the right maxillary sinus (Iconography Di Carlo.R Ref [16]).

6.1.4. Biopsy and Histopathological Study

The biopsy is necessary and obligatory to define the nosological status of any nasosinusal tumors. The biopsy is generally performed under local anesthetic and endoscopic guidance. Multiple biopsies are taken from the periphery and center of the tumor, avoiding necrotic areas. Some endo sinus tumors (without intra-nasal compartment) require a surgical approach for anatomopathological analysis. These surgical biopsies are performed via the middle meatotomy or, more rarely, the vestibular approach.

6.2. Rare and Uncommun Benign Tumor of Maxillary Sinus (Table 9)

Table 9. Rare benign tumor of maxillary sinus [15, 16]

Intra osseous lipoma.
Pleiomorphic adenoma.
Inverted papilloma.
Schwannoma.
Cavernous hemangioma.
Neurofibroma.
Osteoma.
Ameloblastoma.
REHA (respiratory epithelial adenomatoid hamartoma).

6.3. Rare and Uncommun Malignant Tumor of Maxillary Sinus (Table 10)

Table 10. Rare Malignant tumor of maxillary sinus

Esthesioneuroblastoma.
Hodgkin disease of maxillary sinus.
Extra medullary plasmocytoma.
Leiomyosarcoma.
Malignant myoepithelioma.
Myxofibrosarcoma.
Merckel cell carcinoma.
Mucosal malignant melanoma.
Myofibrosarcoma.
Ewing sarcoma.
Intra maxillary sinusal metastatic tumor (esophageal, pulmonary, kidney Breast, Liver).

6.4. Management Principes

The therapeutic management of sinus tumors (benign and malignant) is a difficult task.

The therapeutic management of sinus tumors (benign and malignant) is complex, and relies on the practitioner's experience, a multidisciplinary approach, and expert advice on rare or even exceptional benign and malignant tumor variants. Surgery is the gold standard for the treatment of sinus tumors.

Endoscopic endonasal surgery remains an essential option approach and continues to play an essential role, enabling the patient to undergo surgery under ideal conditions after medium meatotomy and median maxillectomy.

The sheaver, endoscopes 30 and 70, and electric scalpels (monopolar and bipolar) provide surgical comfort.

The histopathological examination of the surgical specimen is a fundamental step towards a definitive diagnosis. Some tumors require additional therapy (radiotherapy, chemotherapy). The follow-up and periodical monitoring is essential, especially for certain tumor types known for their recurrence or metastatic potential.

7. Inflammatory Myofibroblastic (IMT) Tumor of Maxillary Sinus

Inflammatory myofibroblastic tumor (IMT) defined as an intermediate-grade sift tissue myofibroblastic neoplasm by the WHO. In the 2013 classification IMTs are recognized as a clonal neoplasm that are considered to have intermediate malignancy that rarely metastasizes.

7.1. Aetiology

The etiology of IMT is unknown with various report indicating infection or an abnormal immunological reaction. The finding of specific genetic alteration suggests more of a neoplasic etiology than a reactive inflammatory process (Table 11).

Table 11. Pathogenicity of Inflammatory myofibroblastic tumor

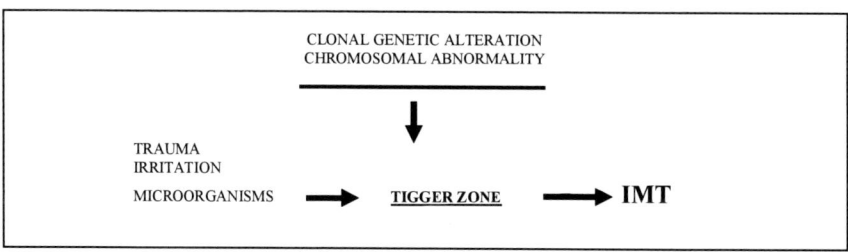

7.2. Diagnosis

The diagnosis of IMT is difficult and cannot be based on clinical findings alone and supplemental histopathological and immunohistochemical studies are necessary. The symptoms are non specific and consist on mass that has been growing over a period of weeks, months or years. The most usually symptom is a local swelling, recurrent and persistent pain.

Imaging is very important from lesion diagnosis, extension, wall destruction, regional scalability, surgical approach, evaluating therapeutic results and follow up. CT scan is the first stapes. CT scan imaging of IMTs in maxillary sinus might be no specific and often suggests infiltrative lesion with aggressive malignant potential (Figure 16). The soft tissue masses in the maxillary sinus is homogeneous without calcification and bone destruction.

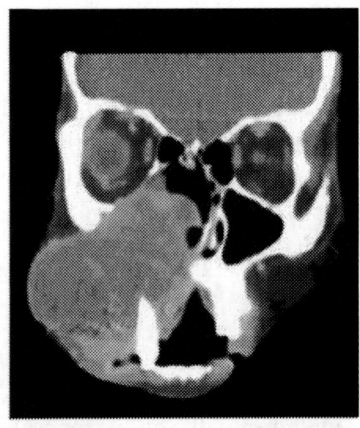

Figure 16. CT Scan coronal incidence: Invasive lesion with highlighting extension (right maxillary sinus) - IMT (Iconography: Hansen.C - Ref: [18]).

MRI indicate size, limits and extension of the tumor. IMT is generally hypodensal in T1 T2 with enhanced after gadolinium. The PET CT (positron emission tomography-computed tomography) is an interesting exam and he reveled the lesion (mass), degree of fixation (SUV) and different locations. It facilitate the evaluation of different modalities of treatment.

Histologically (biopsy or surgical specimen), IMT is composed of admixture of fascicles of myofibroblastic spindle cells with prominent infiltrate of numerous plasma cells, lymphocyes, acute inflammatory cells. The stroma was losse myxoid or edematous. Malignants tumors (myofibroblastic and spindle cell sarcomas) are the principal difficulties to distinguish in IMTs pathology's (Table 12). Immunohistochemistry utilized to confirm the myofibroblastic phenotype of the tumor spindle cells as positive to vimentine, smooth muscle actin, muscle specific actin, desmin, cytokeratine and CD68.IMTs are negative to myoglobine and S-100 protein. ALK-1 test is very important and differentiates IMT from spindle cell neoplasms also referred to as "inflammatory pseudotumors."

Table 12. Inflammatory myofibroblastic tumors: Differential diagnosis

BENIGN TUMORS
Fibromatosis.
Myofibromatosis.
Solitary fibrous tumor.
Benign fibrous histiocytoma.
Wegener's granulomatosis.
MALIGNANT TUMOR
Low-grade myofibroblastic sarcoma.
Malignant fibrous histiocytoma.
Spindle cell carcinoma.
Sarcomatoid carcinoma.
Leiomyosarcoma.
Rhabdomyosarcoma.
Malignant peripheral nerve sheath tumor (MPNST).
Lymphoma.
Plasma cell neoplasms (plasmocytoma, multiple myeloma).

7.3. Therapy

The management of inflammatory myofibroblastic tumors is very difficult and requires necessary a multidisciplinary approach. The therapeutic protocol is chosen after analysis and study of every case between pathologist, surgeon, medical and radiation oncologist practices.

Surgical excision (endoscopic surgery or external approach) with corticosteroid adjuvant therapy is the gold standard and will be chosen in all cases if it is possible.

Radiation therapy (adjunct modality, unresectable and recurrent cases), chemotherapy, and targeted therapy authorize another's opportunities alone or in association. Also we cited NSAIDs, COX2 Inhibitors, tyrosine kinase inhibitors.

7.4. Evolution

The evolution of IMT is unpredictable. It is a severe disease of intermediate malignancy, which may undergo a succession of remissions and recurrences, with locoregional progression to neighboring structures (brain, base of skull, orbits, infra-temporal fossa), resulting in severe functional and structural disorders. Distant metastases and malignant transformations have been reported, further complicating the characteristics of this entity [17]. Some severity criteria have been developed to better define the prognosis of this affection (Table 13). It requires close clinical and imaging follow up (identical to that for cancers), with therapeutic choices being reoriented in response to each new history of the disease.

Table 13. Prognosis factors in inflammatory myofibroblastic tumor (IMT)

TUMOR SIZE.
SURGICAL MARGINS.
ALK-1 LEVELS.
NECROTIC STATUS.
ANATOMIC LOCATION: NASAL AND PARANASAL SITE.

8. Auto Immune Localized Pathology in Maxillary Sinus

8.1. Sarcoidosis Maxillary Sinus

Sarcoidosis is a multisystem granulomatous disease commonly involving the lungs and the mediastinum. This disease affect other organ and extrapulmonary involvement is observed in about 30–40% of patients with sarcoidosis [19, 20].

Bock first reported the sinonasal sarcoidosis in 1905. Sinonasal sarcoidosis is difficult to diagnose and studies estimated that nasal involvement is found in 1–4% of patients with both rhinitis and chronic obstruction.

8.1.1. Aetiology
Saroidosis is a multi-system disease of unknown etiology including genetic susceptibility and environmental factors. The disease characterized by the infiltration of various organ by non necrotizing granulomas.

8.1.2. Diagnosis

Nasal obstruction, rhinorrhea, and chronic sinusitis were the usual initial complaints from patients with maxillary sinus sarcoidosis. Endoscopic exam show mucosal crusting, studding, plaque-like changes, or polyps. Also nasal mucosa present congestion, edematous, hypertrophic or mucosal nodules and in sometime septal perforation.

Radiologic studies showed extensive and often complete opacification of the maxillary sinus and nose similar to that seen in diffuse polyposis associated with chronic bacterial and fungal sinusitis.

PET/CT has the ability to detect FDA uptake in granulomatous cells producing the inflammation seen in sarcoidosis. FDG PET/CT have good sensitivity to evaluate both pulmonary and extra-pulmonary sarcoidosis [21, 22].

Levels of angiotensin-converting enzyme were generally elevated and considered a good and sensible criteria of sarcoidosis diagnosis (Table 14).

We must eliminate differential diagnosis with all diseases with epithelioid granuloma without necrosis (Table 15).

Table 14. Diagnostic criteria for sarcoidosis of the sinuses

1. Radiologic evidence of sinusitis,
2. Histopathologic confirmation of non caseating granuloma in the sinus tissue supported by negative stains for fungus and acid-fast bacilli,
3. Negative serologic test results for syphilis and anti neutrophil cytoplasmic antibodies, and
4. No clinical evidence of other disease processes associated with granulomatous nasal and sinus inflammation (Wegener granulomatosis).
5. Clinical evidence of extra nasal granulomatous (pulmonary) suggesting sarcoidosis.
6. Positive histopathology of salivary accessory gland.
7. 7- Elevated level of angiotensin-converting enzyme

Table 15. Granulomatous diseases

1. Sarcoidosis.
2. Wegener's granulomatosis.
3. Churg-Strauss syndrome.
4. Rheumatoid arthritis.
5. Tuberculosis.
6. Leprosy.
7. Cat-scratch disease.
8. Schistosomiasis.
9. Histiocytosis X.

8.1.3. Therapy
Endoscopic sinus surgery in combination with local intranasal or systemic corticosteroids. Corticosteroids: mean duration of corticosteroid treatment was 3 years, methotrexate, azathioprine, and surgery. TNF-a antagonist adalimumab therapy, leflunomide, chloroquine. An Nasal topical steroid application can help control the progression of isolated nasal involvement.

8.1.4. Evolution
Patients with nasal and paranasal sarcoidosis should be followed carefully over long term by endoscopic exam, angiotensin-converting enzyme level and imaging (Facial CT scan).local recurrence loco-regional progression (orbital, skull base) and systemic involving.

8.2. Auto Immune Diseases and Maxillary Sinus

The nasal mucosa can be a target or an anatomoclinical site for the development and manifestation of symptoms or syndromes associated with autoimmune disease. Thus, the nasosinusal cavities are often affected by lesions and reactions accompanying the onset, development or exacerbation of an autoimmune disease, particularly vasculitis. Knowledge of these manifestations enables early diagnosis (in the case of incipient sinus disease) or provides proof of the nosology of this autoimmune disease (secondary sinus forms), or even medical or surgical intervention to attenuate its effects and improve patients' quality of life.

8.2.1. Symptomatology and Signs of Sinusal Auto Immune Diseases
The clinical rhinologic manifestations of auto immunes diseases are not pathognomonic and needed to observer if we have duration or relapse after every treatment.

Nasal obstruction is habitually and it characterize by progressive beginning unilaterally or with alternance. This obstruction is high in any acute inflammatory access.

Rhinorrhea is very important and constant sign; mucous or mucopurulent type. It attenuates slightly after treatment, but recurs rapidly and becomes more pronounced during inflammatory flare-ups.

Epistaxis is frequent above all in vascularitis disease (Wegener's, Horton, periarteritis nodosa). Nasal bleeding is uni or bilateral, low abundance but recurrent.

Table 16. Connectivits and nasosinusal manifestations

CONNECTIVITIS
RHUMATOID ARTHRITIS.
SYSTEMIC LUPUS ERYTHEMATOSUS.
SCLERODERMIE SYSTEMIQUE.
POLYCHONDRITE ATROPHIQUE.
INFLAMMATORY MYOPATHIES.
GOUGEROT'S-SJOGREN SYNDROME.
ADULT STILL'S DISEASE.
SARCOIDOSIS.
AMYLOSIS.
HYPER IGg-4 RELATED DISEASE.
CLINICS
NASAL OBSTRUCTION, RHNORRHEA, EPISTAXIS, NASAL DEFORMITIES, SEPTAL PERFORATION, DROUGHT HYPOSMIA-ANOSMIA, NASAL CRUSTING.
IMAGING
SINUS OPACITY, HYPERTROPHY SINUSAL MUCOUS, TURBINATES ATROPHIA HYPOPLASIC SINUS, INTRA SINUSAL POLYP.
DIAGNOSIS
BIOLOGY, MUCOSAL BIOPSY, ACCESSORY SALIVARY GLANDES BIOPSY.

Table 17. Vascularitis and nasosinusal manifestations

VASCULARITIS
WEGENER'S POLYANGEITIS
CHURG -STRAUSS SYNDROME
COGAN SYNDROME
HORTON'S DISEASE
PERIARTERITIS NODOSA
KAWASAKI DISEASE
RHUMATOID PURPURA
BEHCET DISEASE
SUSAC SYNDROME
CLINICS
EPISTAXIS, RHIONRRHEA, POLYPOSIS, NASAL OBSTRUCTION, CRUSTING NASAL PERFORATION, INFLAMMATORY MASS, BONE LYSIS, PALATAL PERFORATION TURBINATES NECROSIS.
IMAGING
SINUS OPACITY, HYPERTROPHY SINUSAL MUCOUS, ATROPHIC NASAL LATERAL WALL, HYPOPLASIC SINUS, SINUSES POLYPS.
DIAGNOSIS
BIOLOGY, MUCOSAL BIOPSY, ACCESSORY SALIVARY GLANDES BIOPSY.

Nasal crusting is frequent and associated every time in a lot of auto immune disease (Wegener, sarcoidosis, atrophic polychondritis).

Facial swelling and Pain are frequently observed with any acute inflammatory episode.

Others signs: hyposmia, anosmia, nasal drought (Gougerot-Sjogren disease), palatal perforation (Table 16, 17).

8.2.2. Clinical Diagnosis

The nosological auto immune entity is definite after clinical, imaging and biological screening. Practicien can observing recommendation and criteria of diagnosis about many auto immune disease.

Nasal endoscopy shows congestive and thickness mucosa with secretions and crusting around middle turbinate and meatus. Polyps are frequently observed in some auto immune disease (Churg-Strauss, Sarcoidosis, Rosai-Dorfman disease).

Biology is very important modality of diagnosis and follow up of autoimmune diseases. Laboratory test showed an elevated increased C-reactive protein level, high erythrocyte sedimentation rate and immunological tests.

8.2.3. Therapy

In a few cases, the otorhinolaryngologist can be soliciting in the management of nasosinusal dysfunction in patients who suffer from autoimmune disease. The medical therapy purpose is nasal washing with isotonic serum and a cure of intra-nasal corticosteroids.

In refractory or recurrent rhinosinusitis, polyposis, or complications, a surgical approach by FESS is indicated from amelioration of quality of life.

8.3. Rosai - Dorfman and Maxillary Sinus

Rosai-Dorfman is a rare disease of hematopoietic system and the most common presentation is a painless cervical lymphadenopathy. Paranasal sinus represent one of the two most common extra nodal sites.

8.3.1. Aetiology

The etiology of Rosai-Dorfman disease is unknown and studies have reported a possible relationship with autoimmune diseases, hematological malignancies, post-infectious conditions and immune dysfunction (Table 18).

Table 18. Rosai - Dorfman disease: Pathogenicity

VIRAL INFECTION (EPSTEIN BARR VIRUS, PARVOVIRUS B19, HUMAN HERPES VIRUS). DISORDER OF IMMUNE REGULATION GENETIC MUTATION

8.3.2. Diagnosis

The symptoms of paranasal sinus Rosai-Dorfman location are not specific. Nasal obstruction, rhinorrhea, facial pain, facial swelling, epistaxis, anosmia or hyposmia. We can found also fever, weight loss, night sweats, tonsillitis and cervical lymphadenopathy. Laboratory test showed mild leucocytosis, an elevated increased C-reactive protein level and high erythrocyte sedimentation rate.

CT scan shows homogeneous, hypo intense mass of maxillary sinus with or without extension (orbit, base of skull, inftra temporal fossea). Bone lysis is frequently observed.

In MRI, lesion appear iso dense T1 and heterogeneous T2 (Figure 17, 18).

The PET note an hype metabolism with SUV superior to 13,3 [23].

The diagnosis of Rosai-Dorfman disease was confirmed by histological and immunohistochemical studies. Examination shows multinucleated Langerhans' cells, histiocytes, and eosinophils. Macrophages exhibiting emperipolesis expressing S-100, CD 68, CD19 and CD1 a negative can be considered almost pathognomonic.

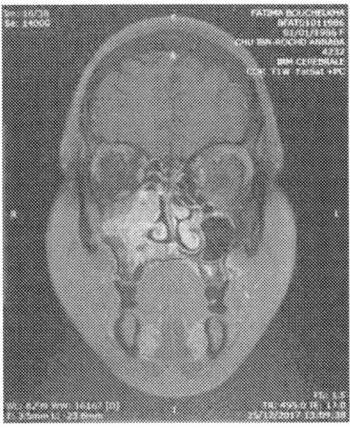

Figure 17. MRI coronal incidence. T2 hyper dense mass occupying left maxillary sinus (Iconography: Kharoubi.s Ref [23]).

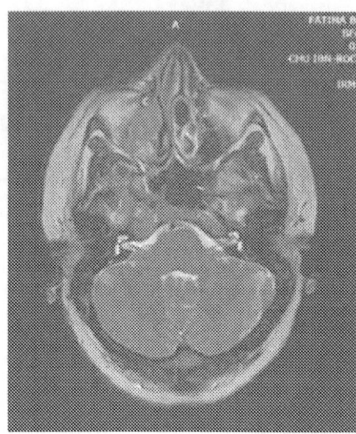

Figure 18. MRI axial incidence. Swelling right part of the face (Iconography: Kharoubi.s Ref [23]).

8.3.3. Therapy

In some cases we can choose abstention and sample following. In 50% of case a treatment was administrated. The surgery is the first line procedure by endoscopic way or external approach. This protocol authorize total or subtotal resection of tumor and histopathological study. Surgery is habitually completed by corticosteroid treatment. Radiation is recommended in relapse or non surgical cases.

Chemotherapy (mercaptopurine, methotrexate, vinblastine, cyclophosphamid) occur a stability of the disease during some weeks or months. Another's modality has been reported like antibiotics, anti fungal agents, acyclovir, diphosphonates, interfron anti-TNF alpha, thalidomide, imatimib.

8.3.4. Evolution

Rosai-Dorfman disease has generally a benign course and is self-limited, it does not require treatment most the time. In a very few cases it may be aggressive course and might be fatal.

The prognosis of Rosai-Dorfman disease is closely linked to the age at onset, involvement of high-risk organs (liver, lung, bone marrow) and response to initial therapy.

9. Foreign Body of the Maxillary Sinus

Foreign bodies are frequently encountered in ENT practice, and are commonly found in the nasal cavities, ears, and pharynx. A foreign body in the paranasal sinuses is rare and 80% of which occur in the maxillary sinus [24].

9.1. Aetiology

There are two main causes of paranasal sinus foreign bodies and it can presented by traumatic or no traumatic causes (Table 19).

1. Non traumatic causes (Iatrogenic or Accidental Foreign bodies): consequence of ENT, ophtalmic and dental procedures and make up 60% of cases [22]. The majority of iatrogenic cases is represented by tooth implant (54%), tooth root and surgical bur [23].
2. Traumatic Foreign bodies: after direct external trauma to the sinus or indirectly through palatal or orbital injuries.

Table 19. Varieties of sinus foreign bodies

DENTAL IMPLANT.
TOOTH ROOTS.
WOODEN STICKS.
TOOTHPICKS.
NEEDLES.
PLASTIC.
GLASS.
MEATAL.
BULLETS.

9.2. Diagnosis

Patients with foreign body in maxillary sinus can present fever, facial pain, headache, nasal obstruction, chronic nasal discharge. In many cases we note total absence of symptoms.

Radiological investigation is the best exam for the diagnosis of paranasal sinus foreign body. Water's radiograph and panoramic view (maxillary sinus) determine the location and content of radiopacity. The CT scan is more accurate that a plain radiograph. CT scan can assess the shape, and exact location of foreign body and is essential in planning the surgical approach. Cone beam computed tomography (CBCT) give good imaging quality and resolution with low radiation exposure.

9.3. Therapy

The treatment of maxillary sinus foreign body is surgical extraction after fine analysis of the location, nature and measurement of the foreign body and the associate lesions (sinusitis) (Table 20). The middle meatal antrostomy is a better technical procedure with low morbidity. The Caldwell Luc procedure is helpful is difficult cases, failure of endoscopic approach or foreign body impacting in anterior wall.

Table 20. Factors to be considerate before removing of paranasal sinus foreign body

- Location.
- Size.
- Shape.
- Composition Of Foreign Body.
- Possibility Of Endoscopic Surgery.
- Foreign Body Associated With Complication.
- (Infection,Perforation,Abcess,Granuloma)
- Mensurations.

10. Maxillary Sinus Rhinolithiasis or Antrolithiasis

Maxillary antrolith are calcified bodies found in the maxillary antrum, know to be formed as the result of mineral salt deposition around a nidus within the antral cavity. The first case has reported by Bowerman in 1969 [26].

10.1. Aetiology

The pathogenesis of antrolith formation is unclear, but we can report long-standing, fungal infection, poor sinus drainage and the presence of foreign body (cotton, paper, dental implants).

10.2. Diagnosis

The diagnosis of antrolithiasis is discovered incidentally on routine radiographic or examinations. Rhinorrhea, nasal obstruction, facial pain, headache, nasal bleeding, chronic sinusitis, oroantral fistula, anosmia, palatal perforation and halitosis can be seen. It is more found commonly in women and young adults [27].

Endonasal endoscopic generally negative or no specific; congestion, secretions, inferior meatus edema, purulent discharge middle meatus. Imaging modalities which can be employed include standard Waters incidence, dental periapical films, panoramic X-rays, CT scan and cone beam (CBCT). Presentation of anthrolith is variable: homogenous or heterogeneous aspect, antral calcification.

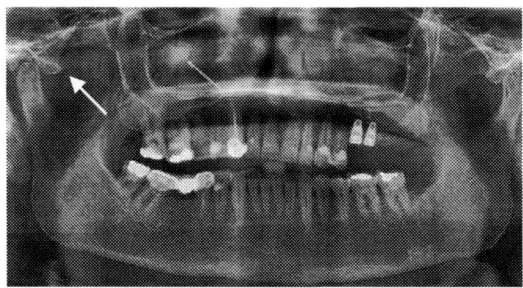

Figure 19. Panoramic X-rays: calcification in right maxillary sinus - antrolithiasis (white arrow) (Iconography: Aoun.G - Ref: [28]).

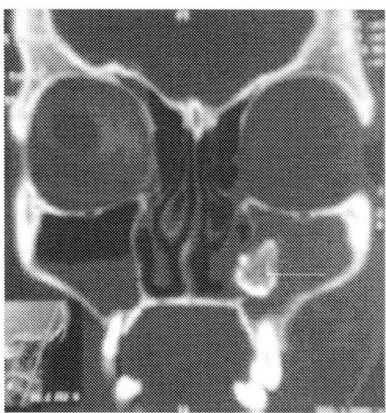

Figure 20. CT Scan coronal incidence: heterogeneous calcification in left maxillary sinus - antrolithiasis (white arrow) (Iconography: Shenoy. V - Ref: [27]).

Table 21. Antrolithiasis: differential diagnosis

Osteomyelitis.
Impacted teeth.
Calcification mucous retention cyst.
Displaced follicular cyst.
Chronic inflammatory processes: tuberculous, syphilis.
Nasal glioma.
Septal dermoid tumor.
Osteoma.
Chondroma.
Calcifying angiofibroma.
Odontoma.
Chondrosarcoma.
Osteosarcoma.

The forms, presentation, localization and mensurations are variables (Figure 19, 20). Imaging also recognize loco regional anomalies (concha bullosa, septal deviation, polyp) and helped differential diagnosis (Table 21).

10.3. Therapy

Surgery is the treatment of choose of antrolithiasis by endoscopic sinus surgery, Caldwell-luc procedure or combination of the two. After removing the antrolith is sended to biochemial analysis (mineral composition).

10.4. Evolution

The prognosis is generally good. Without treatment some complications can involving: infection, fistula, ophthalmic complication, epistaxis, rarely osteomyelitis and epidural abscess [29]. Recurrence is rare.

11. Silent Sinus Syndrome

Silent sinus syndrome (SSS) is a rare disease process characterized by progressive enophtalmos and hypoglobus due to ispilateral maxillary sinus hypoplasia and orbital floor resorption. Its most concern adults but can to be observed in children.

11.1. Aetiology

The etiology remains speculative.

- Pressure theory: (Anomalies of developpement). In this theory during the first or second decade of life, occlusion of the maxillary ostium causes an interruption in normal sinus developpement (Table 22).
- Inflammatory resorption theory: chronic inflammatory could induce erosion of the floor of orbit (elaboration of cytokines).
- Anatomic theory: infection in congenital hypoplastic maxillary sinus.

Table 22. Pressure theory genesis in Silent syndrome sinus

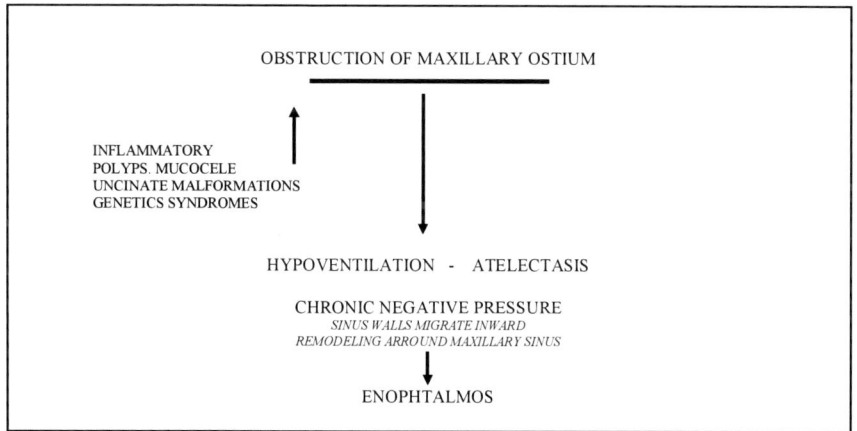

11.2. Diagnosis

Progressive enophtalmos, hypoglobus and asymmetry of the eyes are the principals symptoms to silent sinus syndrome. There are not history of chronic rhinosinusitis is their patients. Along evolution we can noted diplopia and cosmetic deformities.

Endoscopic exam was generally normal or can shows widened middle meatus side with inward retraction of uncinate process.

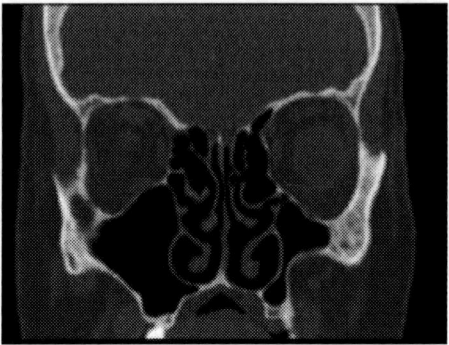

Figure 21. Coronal CT scan. Silent Sinus Syndrome right maxillary sinus (Iconography: Styjewska-Makuch.G - Ref: [30]).

Table 23. Silent sinus syndrome: Differential Diagnosis

HYPOPLASIE MAXILLARY SINUS.
CHRONIC MAXILLARY ATELECTASIS.
TRAUMA OF THE ORBIT.
ORBIT METASTASIS.
WEGENER'S GRANULOMATOSIS.
HIV LIPODYSTROPHY.
ORBITAL FAT ATROPHY.
LINEAR SCLERODERMA.
PSEUDO ENOPHTALMOS.

Histological exam of the mucous of maxillary sinus note chronic inflammation without viable microorganisms.

Coronal CT scans report a reduction of the volume of the maxillary sinus with retraction of all walls of maxillary sinus and augmentation of volume of the orbit. We note also lateralization of uncinate process, expanded middle meatus, deviation of nasal septum and expanded of retroantrum fat pad (Figure 21). Maxillary mucous was thickness. CT scan and MRI facilitate differential diagnosis and follow up of SSS (Table 23).

11.3. Therapy

The management of silent sinus syndrome is surgical. The surgical procedure associate a reconstruction of the orbital floor (titanium mesh implant, autogenous nasal septal cartilage, spilled-thickness bone, auricular concha cartilage) and functional endoscopic sinus surgery (FEES) to remove the obstruction and restore positive pressure.

A single-stage operation is habitually programming (reconstruction of the orbital floor and middle meatotomy) but the orbital floor can to be reconstructed in a late date (six months after FEES) [30]. The surgical treatment is indicate if patients presents severe enophtalmos, diplopia or important facial cosmetic disgrace. A metachronous silent sinus syndrome is possible and has been described in the literature [31].

11.4. Evolution

The observation of ophthalmological signs, in particular severe enophthalmos and diplopia, is an indication for surgery. Surgical results are satisfactory after restoration of maxillary sinus ventilation and reconstruction of the orbital floor. Contralateral involvement remains a possibility.

12. Organising Haematoma of Maxillary Sinus

Organizing haematoma is a rare neoplastic condition witch is locally aggressive.

The first case described is reported in 1917 by Tadokoro as a blood boil of the maxillary sinus [32].

Table 24. Aetiopahogenesis of Organizing haematoma of maxillary sinus

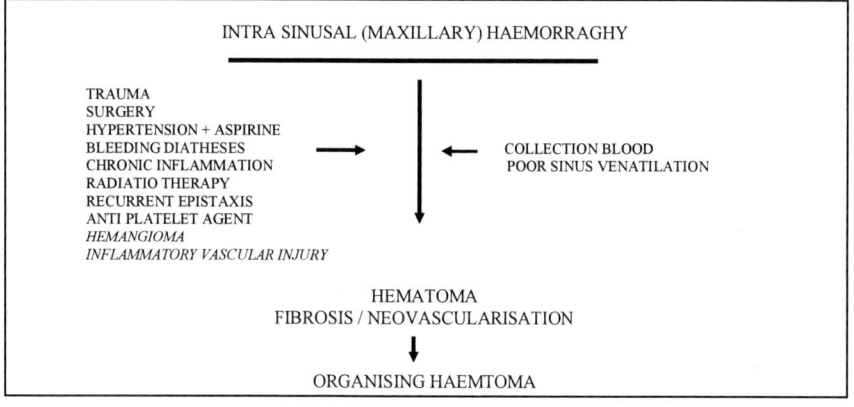

12.1. Aetiology

The first stapes is an maxillary sinus haemorrhagy, formation of hematoma and followed by organization through fibrosis and neovascularisation. Song introduce the terminology of organizing haematoma [33]. The cause of haemorrhagy is unclear but we can found sinus trauma, surgery, hypertension (30% with aspirin), bleeding diatheses (Table 24).

12.2. Diagnosis

Nasal obstruction, rhinorrhea and facial pain are the most symptoms with a normal endonasal exam.

CT scan without contrast shows a large mass causing expansion of the maxillary sinus with bony erosion. Post contrast, patchy heterogeneous enhancement (neovascularization) (Figure 22). On MRI scanning the lesion is heterogeneous in signal intensity on both T1 and T2 [34].

On histological examination organizing hematoma cases snow a combination of vascular ectasia, recent and old hemorrhage, oedema, fibrin exudation, fibrosis and hyalinization and neovascularization.

18FDG-PET shows moderate FDG uptake, the maximum standardized uptake value (SUVmax) of 3,1 to 5,5, only at the periphery of the mass with central photon defects.

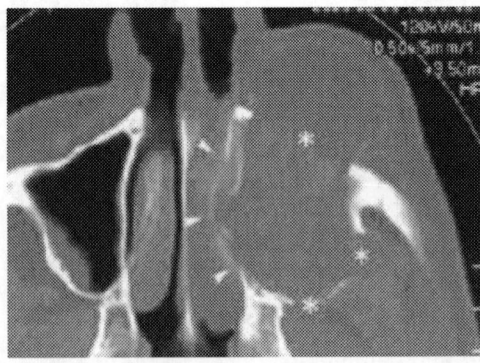

Figure 22. Axial CT scan expanding mass in the left maxillary sinus, medial wall destruction (arrow) and bone defect (asterisks) (Iconography Nishiguchi.T Ref [34]).

12.3. Therapy

The treatment of organizing haematoma is surgical and complete excision. Surgical approach can utilize lateral rhinotomy, Denker's technique's, endoscopic sinus surgery and Caldwell-Luc [35].

12.4. Evolution

Organizing hematoma is rare and can mimic aggressive maxillary sinus tumors. Imaging is helping the diagnosis and the treatment is surgical and consists of complete excision. The recurrence is rare with a good prognosis.

13. Cholesteatoma of the Maxillary Sinus

Cholesteatoma is a condition where respiratory mucosa is replaced by hyperkeratotic squamous epithelium. It was first described by Cruveilhier in 1829.

Haeggstrom reported the first case of cholesteatoma in the frontal sinus (1916).

The first case of maxillary sinus cholesteatoma was reported by Hutcheon (1941).

Cholesteatoma of the maxillary sinus is a rare condition habitually seen in adults but has been described in infants.

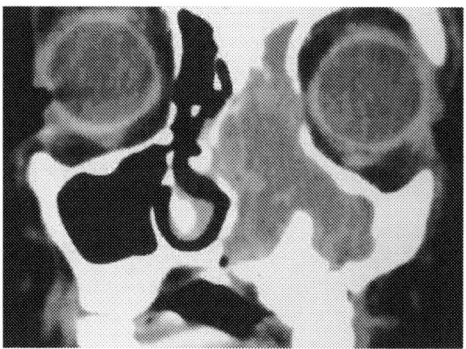

Figure 23. Coronal CTscan: cholesteatoma of the left maxillary sinus. Massin the left nasal cavity with erosion of the lamina papyracea and floor of nasal cavity (Iconography Wishwanata. B Ref [36]).

13.1. Aetiology

- Embryogenic theory: arise from misplaced epithelial rests during embryogenic stage.
- Infection theory: infection induce a metaplastic change of nonkeratizing squamous epithelial lining and produces keratin.
- Migration theory: migration of keratinizing squamous epithelium in an area where it is not usually found.
- Traumatic theory: during previous trauma an after nasal or sinus surgery it arises secondary to the direct entry of epithelium.

13.2. Diagnosis

Symptoms of maxillary sinus cholesteatoma include nasal obstruction, rhinorrhea, facial swelling, exophtalmos or oculo moteur dysfunction and conjonctival oedema. While invasion into the inferior part of the antrum may lead to palate swelling.

The exam of the face shows a tenderness palpation. Endonasal endoscopy revealed that a whitish, friable mass in the nasal cavity and occupied the middle meatus. The biopsy helpful the diagnosis and note hyperkeratotic squamous epithelium [36].

CT scan shows a relativity homogeneous expansile lesion, with osteoclasia in the surrounding area. MRI.

13.3. Therapy

The treatment of maxillary sinus cholesteatoma is surgical by Caldwell- Luc procedure and should be removed entirely to stop further erosion of surrounding structures to prevent recurrence. Endoscopic surgery is also valid and the surgical procedure to cholesteatoma of maxillary sinus should be chosen to allow visibility and complete removal according size, location and extend of disease.

13.4. Evolution

The cholesteatoma of the maxillary sinus grows progressively and procure rhinosinusitis and bone lysis with exteriorization inferior wall (palatal exteriorization) or anterior wall (cheek exteriorization).

OBSERVATION OF CONGENITAL MAXILLARY SINUS CHOLESTEATOMA

Vaz. F has reported one observation of maxillary sinus cholesteatoma in an 18-month-old girl (37).
Symptoms: intra oral and right cheek swelling.
Clinical exam: smooth swelling of the right hard palate in association with the facial swelling in the maxillary region.
Treatment: inferior meatal antrostomy. pultaceous debris in the right maxillary antrum (biopsy confirmed a maxillary sinus cholesteatoma).
Follow up: without recurrence.
Mechanism: congenital cholesteatoma.

Conclusion

The maxillary sinuses, the paranasal cavities, can be the site of many common (rhinosinusitis) or rare, even exceptional, affections. Pathologies of the maxillary sinus can be treated either as isolated primitive conditions, or as manifestations of a general inflammatory or, above all, autoimmune disease. The anatomy of the maxillary sinus makes this approach easy.

Indeed the maxillary sinuses are accessible for clinical (endoscopy) and para-clinical (imaging) exploration, which can help to identify, clarify or control general, metabolic, autoimmune, and tumoral disorders.

The future development of genetics and modern means of exploration (virtual endoscopy, neuro navigation, metabolic imaging, diagnostic cytology) will bring new discoveries and evidence of new pathological entities or diagnostic and therapeutic advances.

References

[1] Neagos A, Dumitru M, Vrinceanu D, Costache A, Marinescu AN, Cergna R Ultrasonography used in the diagnosis of chronic rhinosinusitis: From experimental imaging to clinical pratice. *Experimental and Therapeutic Medicine* 2021 21 611 1-4.

[2] Desal NS, Saboo SS, Ried JA. Pneumosinus dilatans; is it more than an aesthetic concern? *J Craniofac Surg* 2014; 25; 418-21.
[3] Noyek AM, Zizmor J. Pneumocele of the maxillary sinus. *Arch Otolaryngol* 1974; 100 (2): 155-156.
[4] Dilard ML, Sillers MJ. Maxillary sinus pneumocele causing orbital displacement. *Am J Otolaryngol* 1999;20; 250-1.
[5] Jankowski R, Kuntzler S, Boulanger N, Morel O, Tisserant J, Benterkia N, Vignaud JM. Is pneumosinus dilatans an osteogenic disease that mimics the formation of a paranasal sinus ? *Surg Radiol Anat*. 2014; 36; 429-437.
[6] Cho HS, Hong SJ, Chae HK, Kim KS. Maxillary sinus pneumocele presenting as aesthetic deformity: A case report with literature review. *Ear Nose Throat Journal* 2020 Vol 99 (6) 397-401.
[7] Hyun SM, Min JY, Jang YJ. Reduction osteoplasty for treating pneumosinus dilatans of the maxillary sinus. *J Laryngol Otol*, 2013; 127: 207-210.
[8] Choi EC, Shin HS, Nam SM, Park ES, Kim YB. Surgical correction of pneumosinus dilatans of maxillary sinus. *J Craniofac Surg* 2011,22: 978-981.
[9] Kukreja HK, Sacha BS, Joshi KC. Tuberculosis of the maxillary sinus. *Indian J Otolaryngol* 1977 29 27.
[10] Beltran S, Douadi Y, Lescure FX, Hanau M, Laurans G, Ducrois JP. A case of tuberculous sinusitis without concomitant pulmonary disease. *Eur J Clin Microbiol Infect Dis* 2003; 22: 49-50.
[11] Sanehi S, Dravid C, Chaudhary N, Venkatachalam VP. Tuberculosis of paranasal sinuses. *Indian J Otolaryngol Head Neck Surg*. 2008 Mar;60(1):85-7. doi: 10.1007/s12070-008-0027-8.
[12] Rayapati DK, Prashanth NT, Rangan V, Kalakunta PR. Tuberculosis of the maxillary sinus masquerading as a facial abscess, a unique occurrence. *J Oral Maxillofac Pathol*. 2018 Jan; 22 (Suppl 1): S126-S130. doi: 10.4103/jomfp.JOMFP_119_16.
[13] Gilmore A, Roller J, Dyer JA Leprosy (Hansen's disease): An update and review. *Missouri Medicine* January/February 2023 120;1 39-44.
[14] Maymone M, Venkatesh S, Laughter M, and Al Leprosy: treatment and management of complications. *J Am Acad Dermatol* 2020 83 17-30.
[15] Uysal A, Kayiran O, Cuzdan SS, Bektas CI, Aslan G, Caydere M. Maxillary sinus lipoma: an unanticipated diagnosis. *J Craniofac Surg*. 2007 Sep;18(5):1153-5. doi: 10.1097/scs.0b013e3180f61262.
[16] Di Carlo R, Rinaldi R, Ottaviano G, Pastore A. Respiratory epithelial adenomatoid hamartoma of the maxillary sinus: case report. *Acta Otorhinolaryngol Ital*. 2006 Aug;26(4):225-7.
[17] Saiji E, Guillou L. Fibroblastic and myofibroblastic tumors of the head and neck. *Ann Pathol* 2009 29 335-346.
[18] Hansen CC, Eisenbach C, Torres C, Graham S, Hardwicke F Maxillary sinus inflammatory myofibroblastic tumors: A review and case report. *Case reports in Oncological Medecine*. Volume 2015 doi/10.1155/2015/953857.

[19] Rybicki BA, Major M, Popovich J Jr, Maliarik MJ, Iannuzzi MC. Racial differences in sarcoidosis incidence: A 5-year study in a health maintenance organization. *Am J Epidemiol* 1997, 145:234–241.
[20] Rajeh A, Albers A, Pudszuhn A, Hofmann VM. Rare involvement of paranasal sinuses in sarcoidosis: case report and literature review. *Pan Afr Med J.* 2019 Jul 24;33:250. doi: 10.11604/pamj.2019.33.250.16922.
[21] Signore A, Glaudemans AW. The molecular imaging approach to image infections and inflammation by nuclear medicine techniques. *Ann Nucl Med* 2011; 25 : 681-700.
[22] Kung TB, Seraj SM, Zadeh MZ, Rojulpote C, Kothekar E, Ayubcha C and Al An update on the role of ^{18}F-FDG-PET/CT in major infectious and inflammatory diseases. *Am J Nucl Med Mol Imaging.* 2019 Dec 15;9(6):255-273.
[23] Kharoubi S. Rosai-Dorfman disease of maxillary sinus. Presse medicale 2019 Tome 48 N°3 mars 333-335.
[24] Agarwal S, Kumar S. Foreign bodies in maxillary sinus: Causes and management. *Astrocyte* 2014, 1 (2): 89-92.
[25] Deniz Y, Zengin AZ, Karli R. An unusual foreign body in the maxillary sinus: dental impression material. *Niger J Clin Pract,* 2016; 19 (2) : 298-300.
[26] Bowerman JE. The maxillary antrolith. *J Laryngo Otol* 1969 83 873-882.
[27] Shenoy V, Maller V, Maller V. Maxillary antrolith: a rare cause of the recurrent sinusitis. *Case reports in Otolaryngology* Vol 2013 Article ID 527152 4 pages. doi.org/10.1155/2013/527152.
[28] Aoun G, Nasseh I. Maxillary antroliths: a digital panoramic-based study. *Cureus* 12 (1) 1-6 e 6686. doi: 10.7759/cureus.6686.
[29] Singh R, Varshney S, Bist S, Gupta N, Bhatia R, Kishore S. Rhinolithiasis and value of nasal endoscopy: a case report. J Otorhnolaryngol 2007 7.
[30] Stryjewska-Makuch G, Goroszkiewicz K, Szymocha J, Lisowska G, Misiołek M. Etiology, Early Diagnosis and Proper Treatment of Silent Sinus Syndrome Based on Review of the Literature and Own Experience. *J Oral Maxillofac Surg.* 2022 Jan;80(1):113.e1-113.e8. doi: 10.1016/j.joms.2021.08.166.
[31] Babar-Craig H, Kayhanian H, De silva DJ, Rose GE, Lund VJ. Spontaneaous silent syndrome (imploding antrum syndrome): case series of 16 patients. *Rhinology* 2011; 49 : 315-317.
[32] Farneti P, Bellusci A, Parmeggiani A, Pasquini E. Metachronous Bilateral Silent Sinus Syndrome: A Case Report. *Iran J Otorhinolaryngol.* 2020 May;32(110):175-179. doi: 10.22038/ijorl.2020.42809.2396.
[33] Tadokoro K. *Jyougakudou Ketsurryu ni tsuite [About the maxillary sinus] Dainichi Jibi [Dainichi ear nose]* 1917; 23: 359-360.
[34] Song HM, Jang YJ, Chung YS, Lee BJ. Organizing hematoma of the maxillary sinus. Otolaryngol Head Neck Surg 2007 136 616-620.
[35] Nishiguchi T, Nakamura A, Mochuziki K, Tokuhara Y, Yamane H, Inoue Y. Expansile organized maxillary sinus hematoma: MR and CT findings and review of literature. *AJNR Am J Neuroradiol* Aug 2007 28: 1375-77.
[36] Yasigawa M, Ishitoya J, Tsukuda M. Hematoma-like mass of the maxillary sinus. *Acta Otolaryngol* 2006; 126: 277-281.

[37] Viswanatha B. Cholesteatoma of the nose and maxillary and ethmoid sinuses: A rare complication of palatal surgery. *Ent-Ear, Nose and Throat Journal*. Septembre 2011 428-430.
[38] Vaz F, Callanan V, Leighton S, Risdon RA. Congenital maxillary sinus cholesteatoma. *Int J Pediatr Otorhinolaryngol.* 2000 May 30;52(3):283-6. doi: 10.1016/s0165-5876(00)00289-5.

Chapter 2

Odontogenic-Related Maxillary Sinusitis: Unraveling Microbial Dynamics and Preventive Strategies in Multidisciplinary Care

Hema Suryawanshi[1] and Santosh R. Patil[2,*]

[1]Department of Oral Pathology and Microbiology,
Chhattisgarh Dental College & Research Institute, India,
[2]Department of Oral Medicine and Radiology,
Chhattisgarh Dental College & Research Institute, India

Abstract

Maxillary sinusitis originating from dental issues poses a unique and intricate challenge in clinical practice. This chapter delves into the complex interplay between acute and chronic maxillary sinusitis and odontogenic factors, elucidating the microbiological underpinnings crucial for effective prevention and management. By exploring the microbial profile associated with acute and chronic cases, this chapter aims to enhance our understanding of the etiological factors involved in odontogenic-related maxillary sinusitis.

The focus then shifts to preventive measures, encompassing both individual responsibilities and the pivotal role of dental professionals. Emphasis is placed on the significance of optimal oral hygiene practices as a fundamental line of defense against bacterial or fungal colonization that may contribute to sinus infections. Antimicrobial mouthwashes, tongue cleaning, and daily oral care routines are discussed as essential components of a proactive approach to mitigate the risk of sinusitis.

---

[*] Corresponding Author's Email: drpsantosh@gmail.com.

In: Maxillary Sinus Diseases
Editor: Anisha Webb
ISBN: 979-8-89113-534-5
© 2024 Nova Science Publishers, Inc.

Furthermore, the chapter highlights the crucial role of regular dental check-ups in preventing odontogenic-related maxillary sinusitis. Dental professionals are positioned to identify and address dental issues early on, preventing the progression of infections to the maxillary sinus. Timely intervention, patient education, and post-operative care instructions following dental procedures are essential components of this preventive strategy. This chapter also serves as a comprehensive guide for clinicians, researchers, and dental healthcare providers involved in the multidisciplinary care of individuals at risk for odontogenic-related maxillary sinusitis. By elucidating the microbial landscape and emphasizing preventive strategies, it aims to contribute to the enhancement of patient outcomes and the overall management of this intricate clinical entity.

Keywords: maxillary sinusitis, odontogenic origin, microbiology, dental infections oral hygiene, multidisciplinary care

Introduction

Maxillary sinusitis, a prevalent medical condition characterized by inflammation of the maxillary sinus, holds significant clinical ramifications. Nestled within the maxillary bone, the maxillary sinus plays a pivotal role in the intricate balance of the upper respiratory system. The repercussions of its inflammation are manifested through a spectrum of symptoms, ranging from facial pain and nasal congestion to persistent headaches (Bell et al., 2011). This introductory exploration seeks to underscore the critical importance of understanding the etiological factors behind maxillary sinusitis for efficacious diagnostic strategies and treatment modalities.

A noteworthy facet of maxillary sinusitis lies in its association with odontogenic issues. The intimate proximity of the maxillary sinus to dental structures establishes a potential conduit for the transmission of infections from the oral cavity to the sinus. This dynamic connection underscores the symbiotic relationship between oral health and sinus conditions, necessitating a meticulous examination of the microbiological intricacies involved (Psillas et al., 2021).

Microbiology emerges as the linchpin in unraveling the multifaceted nature of maxillary sinusitis. The identification of specific microbial agents responsible for sinus infections stands as a pivotal step in tailoring targeted therapeutic interventions. Within this framework, the convergence of odontogenic issues and maxillary sinusitis introduces an additional layer of complexity to the microbial landscape. Consequently, a nuanced understanding becomes imperative for clinicians to navigate this intricate terrain effectively (Brook, 2005).

As we embark on a comprehensive exploration of the microbiology inherent in maxillary sinusitis associated with an odontogenic origin, the need for a thorough examination of microbial profiles becomes self-evident. This chapter endeavors to offer an in-depth analysis of the diverse microbial agents intricately linked to acute and chronic maxillary sinusitis, particularly those stemming from dental sources. Through this exploration, our aim is to enrich the medical community's comprehension of the subtleties surrounding odontogenic-related maxillary sinusitis. By doing so, we aspire to contribute to heightened diagnostic precision and improved treatment outcomes, thus advancing the collective knowledge and clinical approach to this intriguing facet of sinus pathology.

Anatomy of the Maxillary Sinus

The maxillary sinus, one of the four paired paranasal sinuses, is a pyramidal-shaped cavity located within the maxillary bone. Positioned laterally to the nasal cavity, it plays a crucial role in various physiological functions, such as humidification and filtration of inhaled air. The floor of the maxillary sinus corresponds to the alveolar process of the maxilla, which contains the upper teeth, particularly the premolars and molars (Iwanga et al., 2019).

The proximity of the maxillary sinus to dental structures is of significant clinical relevance. The roots of the maxillary posterior teeth can extend in close proximity to the sinus floor, creating an anatomical relationship that has implications for both dental and sinus health. The most common area of proximity is the region of the maxillary molars, where the roots may be in direct contact with the sinus floor or even project into the sinus space (Iwanga et al., 2019).

This close association between dental structures and the maxillary sinus introduces the potential for communication between these two anatomical regions. Pathological conditions affecting the teeth, such as infections or dental procedures, can lead to the spread of infections to the adjacent sinus. This phenomenon is particularly relevant when exploring the odontogenic origin of maxillary sinusitis, where microbial agents from dental sources may play a crucial role in the initiation and progression of sinus infections (Gosau et al., 2009).

Understanding the anatomical relationship between the maxillary sinus and dental structures is paramount for healthcare professionals in various fields, including dentistry, otolaryngology, and infectious disease, as it forms the basis for comprehending the potential pathways through which odontogenic factors can contribute to sinusitis. This knowledge is crucial for accurate diagnosis and effective management of maxillary sinusitis associated with dental issues (Davis et al., 1996)

Etiology of Maxillary Sinusitis

Maxillary sinusitis is a prevalent condition that can arise from various etiological factors, encompassing bacterial, viral, and fungal agents. Understanding the diverse contributors to sinusitis is essential for accurate diagnosis and effective management.

Common Bacterial Causes

Bacterial infections are among the leading causes of maxillary sinusitis. Streptococcus pneumoniae and Haemophilus influenzae are frequently implicated in acute cases. Additionally, Staphylococcus aureus, including methicillin-resistant strains, has been identified in both acute and chronic maxillary sinusitis cases (DeBoer et al., 2023).

Viral Agents

Viruses, particularly respiratory viruses, play a significant role in the etiology of acute maxillary sinusitis. Common culprits include rhinoviruses, influenza viruses, and adenoviruses. Viral infections often predispose individuals to secondary bacterial infections, further complicating the clinical picture (Puhakka 1998).

Fungal Involvement

Fungal sinusitis is another subset of maxillary sinusitis, with different forms such as allergic fungal sinusitis and invasive fungal sinusitis. Aspergillus species are commonly associated with fungal sinus infections, particularly in immunocompromised individuals (Akhondi et al., 2023).

Odontogenic Factors

An intriguing aspect of maxillary sinusitis is its association with odontogenic factors. Dental infections, particularly those involving the upper molars, can lead to the spread of pathogens from dental structures to the maxillary sinus. Periapical abscesses and dental granulomas can serve as reservoirs for bacteria, facilitating their migration to the sinus cavity (Mehra et al., 2099).

Role of Odontogenic Factors

Odontogenic sources contribute to sinusitis through several mechanisms. The proximity of dental roots to the floor of the maxillary sinus provides an anatomical pathway for bacterial migration. Inflammatory processes within dental tissues, such as pulpitis or periodontal disease, can result in the release of infectious agents into the sinus cavity (Mehra et al., 2099).

Furthermore, dental procedures, such as extractions or root canal treatments, carry a risk of introducing bacteria into the sinus, especially if the Schneiderian membrane is compromised during the procedure. Chronic odontogenic infections may lead to persistent or recurrent maxillary sinusitis, emphasizing the importance of considering dental health in the assessment of sinusitis cases (Kim, 2019).

In summary, maxillary sinusitis is a multifaceted condition with diverse etiological factors, encompassing bacterial, viral, and fungal agents. Odontogenic factors, in particular, play a crucial role in the development and perpetuation of sinusitis, highlighting the interconnectedness of oral and sinus health. A comprehensive understanding of these etiological factors is essential for devising effective diagnostic and therapeutic strategies in the management of maxillary sinusitis.

Microbial Pathogens in Acute Maxillary Sinusitis

Acute maxillary sinusitis is a common condition marked by the rapid onset of inflammation within the maxillary sinus, primarily triggered by microbial infections. A deeper exploration into the microbial profile associated with this ailment is pivotal for enhancing diagnostic accuracy and tailoring effective treatment strategies. Recent investigations have significantly contributed to our understanding of the specific bacteria, viruses, and fungi implicated in acute cases, providing nuanced insights into the intricate etiology of this prevalent sinus disorder.

1. *Bacterial Agents*: Bacterial involvement is paramount in the pathogenesis of acute maxillary sinusitis. Key bacterial pathogens frequently identified in acute cases include Streptococcus pneumoniae, Haemophilus influenzae, and Moraxella catarrhalis. These bacteria are part of the normal flora inhabiting the upper respiratory tract, but under certain conditions, they transition to opportunistic pathogens, instigating sinus infections. The prevalence of these bacterial species exhibits geographical and demographic variations, influencing the clinical manifestation of acute maxillary sinusitis (Swada, 2021).
2. *Viral Infections*: Beyond bacterial contributions, viral infections significantly contribute to the complexity of acute maxillary sinusitis, often acting in synergy with bacterial agents. Recent research underscores the involvement of respiratory viruses such as rhinovirus, influenza virus, and adenovirus in exacerbating sinusitis symptoms. The intricate interplay between viral and bacterial pathogens not only complicates clinical presentations but also extends the duration of symptoms, emphasizing the imperative role of precise diagnosis for optimal therapeutic interventions (Boncristiani et al., 2009).
3. *Fungal Infections*: Although less common, fungal infections should not be disregarded, particularly in immunocompromised individuals. Aspergillus species, known for their association with fungal sinusitis, can invade the sinus cavity, leading to a more severe and chronic course of the disease (Peral-Cagigal et al., 2014). Recognizing fungal involvement is crucial for tailoring antifungal therapies when necessary, preventing the progression of the infection.
4. Advancements in Microbial Characterization: Recent studies have harnessed advanced molecular techniques to characterize the

microbial landscape in acute maxillary sinusitis more comprehensively. High-throughput sequencing technologies have enabled a more in-depth identification of microbial communities, providing insights into the role of the microbiome in sinusitis pathogenesis (Abreu et al., 2012). Such studies reveal the complexity of microbial interactions in acute cases, emphasizing the need for personalized treatment approaches based on the specific microbial profile of each patient.

In conclusion, acute maxillary sinusitis presents as a multifaceted condition with a diverse microbial etiology. The intricate interplay of bacterial, viral, and fungal pathogens underscores the complexity of this ailment. Recent advancements in molecular techniques not only enhance our understanding of the microbial landscape associated with acute sinusitis but also pave the way for more targeted and effective therapeutic strategies.

Microbial Pathogens in Chronic Maxillary Sinusitis

Chronic maxillary sinusitis, characterized by persistent inflammation of the maxillary sinuses lasting more than 12 weeks, represents a multifaceted condition influenced by a diverse range of microbial pathogens. The intricate interplay of bacteria, viruses, and fungi contributes to the chronicity of the disease, making a comprehensive understanding of the microbial profile imperative for effective diagnosis and treatment.

Bacterial Infections

Bacterial involvement in chronic maxillary sinusitis is well-documented, with certain species demonstrating a predilection for persisting infections. Among these, Staphylococcus aureus, particularly methicillin-resistant strains (MRSA), has been prominently identified in chronic cases (Rujanavej et al., 2013). This prevalence of MRSA adds a layer of complexity to treatment strategies, as these strains often exhibit resistance to conventional antibiotics. Additionally, gram-positive bacteria like Streptococcus pneumoniae and anaerobic bacteria, including Prevotella and Fusobacterium species, contribute to the microbial consortium in chronic sinusitis (Fastenberg et al., 2016). The formation of biofilms by these bacteria on the sinus mucosa poses a significant challenge, as these structures provide a protective environment, hindering the efficacy of antibiotic therapy (Fastenberg et al., 2016)

Viral Infections

Traditionally associated with acute sinusitis, viral infections have been increasingly recognized as contributors to the chronic variant. Human rhinovirus and influenza viruses have been detected in the sinuses of patients with chronic maxillary sinusitis, indicating a potential ongoing viral contribution to the inflammatory process (Jacobs et al., 2013). The interaction between viral and bacterial agents within the sinus mucosa adds an additional layer of complexity to the microbial landscape in chronic cases, influencing the persistence and exacerbation of symptoms.

Fungal Infections

Fungal infections, particularly those caused by molds, have emerged as significant contributors to chronic maxillary sinusitis. Aspergillus species, notably Aspergillus fumigatus, have been identified in sinus samples, particularly in individuals with underlying immunocompromised conditions (Bandres et al., 2023). Fungal infections may intensify the inflammatory response and complicate treatment approaches, necessitating antifungal therapy in conjunction with antibacterial agents to address the multifactorial nature of chronic sinusitis.

In summary, chronic maxillary sinusitis is intricately linked to a diverse microbial profile involving bacteria, viruses, and fungi. A nuanced understanding of the specific pathogens and their interactions is crucial for tailoring effective therapeutic strategies and addressing the persistent and complex nature of this condition.

Odontogenic Origin of Sinusitis

Maxillary sinusitis originating from dental sources, known as odontogenic sinusitis, results from the spread of infections from the oral cavity to the maxillary sinus. This section delves into the intricate relationship between dental structures and the maxillary sinus, exploring the pathways of infection, microbial pathogens involved, and the diagnostic and therapeutic considerations.

Dental Contributions to Maxillary Sinusitis

The anatomical proximity of the maxillary sinus to the upper teeth allows for the direct extension of infections from dental structures into the sinus cavity. Dental caries, periapical abscesses, and periodontal diseases can serve as sources of odontogenic sinusitis. The initiation of odontogenic sinusitis often involves bacterial infiltration from infected dental pulp into the surrounding periapical tissues (Psillas et al., 2021). In particular, molars, with their extensive root systems, are commonly associated with odontogenic sinusitis.

Microbial Pathogens in Odontogenic Sinusitis

The microbiology of odontogenic sinusitis involves a diverse array of bacteria commonly found in the oral cavity. Studies have consistently identified Streptococcus species, Prevotella, Fusobacterium, and various anaerobic bacteria as prevalent in odontogenic sinus infections (Little, 2018). These organisms may gain access to the maxillary sinus through periapical lesions, dental caries, or breaches in the bone surrounding tooth roots.

Clinical Evidence Supporting Odontogenic Origin

Clinical evidence supports the association between dental pathologies and sinus infections. Imaging studies, such as cone-beam computed tomography (CBCT), have played a pivotal role in establishing these connections. These advanced imaging techniques reveal the intricate relationship between dental structures and the maxillary sinus, highlighting periapical lesions, dental abscesses, and communication channels between the oral cavity and the sinus (Peñarrocha-Oltra et al., 2020).

Pathways of Infection

The pathways through which odontogenic infections reach the maxillary sinus are multifaceted. In the case of periapical lesions, bacteria from an infected tooth's root apex can extend into the adjacent maxillary bone, providing a direct route to the sinus cavity (Hauman, 2002). Similarly, periodontal diseases, such as periodontitis, can create pathways for bacterial migration from the oral cavity to the sinus, contributing to the development of odontogenic sinusitis (Psillas et al., 2021).

Diagnosing odontogenic sinusitis requires a comprehensive approach that includes clinical evaluation, imaging, and microbial analysis. CBCT scans are particularly valuable in identifying dental pathologies and their relationship with sinus inflammation. Clinical symptoms such as dental pain, purulent nasal discharge, and tenderness over the maxillary sinuses are essential diagnostic indicators. Microbial analysis through culture or molecular methods aids in identifying the specific pathogens involved, guiding targeted antimicrobial therapy (Craig et al., 2021). Once diagnosed, management involves addressing the underlying dental issues. Root canal therapy, tooth extraction, or periodontal treatment may be necessary to eliminate the source of infection. Concurrently, antimicrobial therapy directed against the identified pathogens is crucial for effective resolution. Surgical intervention may be considered in cases where there is persistent infection or complications such as abscess formation.

In summary, odontogenic sinusitis represents a distinct form of maxillary sinusitis with origins in dental structures. The interplay between oral health and sinus health is evident, with dental infections serving as a potential source of sinus inflammation. Understanding the microbial profile associated with odontogenic sinusitis, along with advancements in diagnostic imaging, allows for targeted therapeutic interventions, ensuring comprehensive management of this specific form of maxillary sinusitis.

Diagnostic Approaches

Accurate diagnosis of maxillary sinusitis associated with an odontogenic origin is paramount for effective treatment strategies. Several diagnostic methods contribute to a comprehensive understanding of the microbial pathogens involved in sinus infections.

Imaging Techniques
Radiological imaging stands as a pivotal diagnostic tool for maxillary sinusitis. High-resolution computed tomography (HRCT) scans provide intricate details of the sinus anatomy, enabling clinicians to identify structural abnormalities, mucosal thickening, and the presence of fluid indicative of sinusitis (Yoshiura et al., 1993). In cases linked to odontogenic factors, dental cone-beam computed tomography (CBCT) emerges as particularly valuable, offering detailed views of dental structures and their relationship to the maxillary sinus (Bromberg et al., 2023). Imaging aids in differentiating between acute and chronic sinusitis, guiding clinicians in determining the extent of the infection and potential sources, including dental origins.

Cultural Methods
Traditional cultural techniques involve the isolation and identification of microbial agents from clinical samples, typically obtained through sinus puncture and aspiration. While invasive, these methods remain the gold standard for obtaining reliable cultures directly from the sinus cavity. Common bacterial pathogens isolated in acute maxillary sinusitis cases include Streptococcus pneumoniae, Haemophilus influenzae, and Moraxella catarrhalis (Mahdavinia et al., 2016). However, cultural methods may have limitations, such as potential contamination and difficulty obtaining samples from chronic cases, highlighting the need for complementary diagnostic approaches.

Molecular Techniques
Advancements in molecular diagnostics have revolutionized the precision and speed of identifying microbial pathogens. Polymerase chain reaction (PCR) assays targeting specific microbial DNA/RNA sequences enable the detection of bacteria, viruses, and fungi with high sensitivity and specificity (Badiee et al., 2015). Molecular techniques are particularly advantageous in cases where traditional culture methods may fail to identify fastidious or uncultivable pathogens. They also allow for the simultaneous detection of multiple pathogens in a single sample, facilitating a more comprehensive understanding of the microbial profile in sinusitis cases.

Challenges in Accurate Diagnosis
Despite the arsenal of diagnostic tools available, challenges persist in achieving accurate and timely diagnoses. The polymicrobial nature of

odontogenic sinusitis, with diverse bacterial species often coexisting, poses challenges in isolating and identifying all relevant pathogens. Furthermore, biofilm formation within the sinus cavity can hinder the effectiveness of traditional cultural methods, making it difficult to obtain accurate microbial profiles (Areizaga-Madina et al., 2023). In chronic cases, the intermittent nature of symptoms and the potential for low-grade infections may further complicate diagnosis.

Integration of Diagnostic Methods
Given the challenges, a comprehensive diagnostic approach integrating imaging, cultural, and molecular techniques is essential. Imaging provides a visual roadmap, guiding subsequent diagnostic steps. Cultural methods offer direct evidence of pathogens but may be limited in chronic cases. Molecular techniques bridge these gaps, offering rapid and specific identification, particularly useful when dealing with complex, polymicrobial infections. The integration of these diagnostic methods enhances the accuracy of identifying microbial pathogens, guiding clinicians in developing targeted and effective treatment plans.

In summary, the diagnostic landscape for maxillary sinusitis associated with an odontogenic origin involves a combination of imaging, cultural, and molecular techniques. Each method contributes unique insights, and their integration is essential for overcoming the challenges posed by the complex microbiology of sinusitis, allowing for more precise and tailored treatment strategies.

Treatment Strategies

Maxillary sinusitis, whether acute or chronic, necessitates a comprehensive treatment strategy that combines antimicrobial therapy, the resolution of underlying odontogenic issues, and, when necessary, surgical interventions. This multifaceted approach is crucial for achieving effective management and preventing recurrence.

Antimicrobial Therapy for Acute and Chronic Cases

Antimicrobial therapy is a cornerstone in the treatment of maxillary sinusitis, aiming to eradicate microbial pathogens causing the infection. In acute cases, early initiation of antibiotics is crucial. Common pathogens include Streptococcus pneumoniae, Haemophilus influenzae, and Moraxella catarrhalis. Empirical treatment often involves broad-spectrum antibiotics such as amoxicillin-clavulanate, with adjustments based on culture and sensitivity results (Al-Saadi, 2018).

Addressing Underlying Odontogenic Issues

The successful management of maxillary sinusitis requires a thorough investigation and resolution of underlying odontogenic factors. Dental issues, including periapical abscesses or periodontal disease, can serve as reservoirs for infection, perpetuating sinusitis. Collaboration between otolaryngologists and dental professionals is crucial for a comprehensive treatment plan.

Root canal therapy, tooth extraction, or periodontal interventions may be necessary to eliminate the source of infection. The involvement of dental specialists ensures a targeted approach to address odontogenic contributions, thereby reducing the risk of recurrent sinusitis. This collaborative effort is essential for identifying and managing dental factors that may otherwise be overlooked in a solely medical approach (Kim, 2019).

Surgical Interventions

When antimicrobial therapy and addressing odontogenic issues prove insufficient, surgical interventions become a pivotal aspect of the treatment strategy. Functional endoscopic sinus surgery (FESS) is commonly employed for chronic cases, allowing direct visualization and drainage of the sinuses. FESS also provides access to the odontogenic region for necessary dental procedures (Al-Mujaini et al., 2009).

The decision to pursue surgical intervention is guided by the severity and chronicity of symptoms, as well as the response to initial medical treatments. Surgical intervention becomes integral in cases where anatomical or structural abnormalities contribute to persistent or recurrent sinusitis.

In summary, an integrated approach to maxillary sinusitis involves not only antimicrobial therapy tailored to the specific microbial profile but also the identification and resolution of underlying odontogenic issues. Surgical interventions, particularly FESS, play a crucial role in cases resistant to conservative measures. A collaborative effort between medical and dental professionals ensures a comprehensive and patient-centered treatment plan, minimizing the risk of recurrence and optimizing long-term outcomes.

Preventive Measures

Preventing odontogenic-related maxillary sinusitis is crucial for maintaining overall oral and sinus health. A combination of good oral hygiene practices and regular dental check-ups plays a pivotal role in minimizing the risk of infection and subsequent sinus complications.

Below table provides a summary of the key points from the two sections on Preventive Measures for Odontogenic-Related Maxillary Sinusitis

Preventive Measures

Oral Hygiene Practices	Encourage comprehensive oral care routines to reduce bacterial or fungal colonization.
	Emphasize daily brushing and flossing to remove dental plaque as a reservoir for potential pathogens.
	Recommend antimicrobial mouthwashes, especially those with chlorhexidine, for reducing bacterial load.
	Educate individuals on proper tongue cleaning to contribute to a healthier oral microbiome.
Regular Dental Check-ups	Highlight the pivotal role of dentists in early detection and intervention for dental issues.
	Emphasize prompt treatment for dental infections to prevent their spread to adjacent structures.
	Provide post-operative care instructions, especially for dental procedures with a risk of sinus involvement.
	Educate patients about signs and symptoms of dental infections to promote timely dental care seeking.

Conclusion

The exploration of odontogenic-related maxillary sinusitis in this manuscript underscores the intricate interplay between oral health and sinus conditions, shedding light on microbial dynamics, preventive strategies, and the importance of multidisciplinary care. The anatomical proximity of dental structures to the maxillary sinus establishes a potential pathway for infections, emphasizing the need for a nuanced understanding of etiological factors.

Microbiology stands as a linchpin in unraveling the complexities of maxillary sinusitis, with bacterial, viral, and fungal agents contributing to both acute and chronic cases. The association of odontogenic factors introduces an additional layer of intricacy, highlighting the interconnectedness of oral and sinus health. Advances in diagnostic techniques, including imaging, cultural, and molecular methods, enable a more precise identification of microbial pathogens, guiding targeted therapeutic interventions.

Preventive strategies, ranging from optimal oral hygiene practices to regular dental check-ups, form a crucial line of defense against odontogenic-related maxillary sinusitis. Emphasizing patient education and post-operative care instructions adds a proactive dimension to prevention. Multidisciplinary care, involving collaboration among healthcare professionals, ensures a comprehensive approach to diagnosis, treatment, and ongoing management.

The multidimensional nature of odontogenic-related maxillary sinusitis necessitates ongoing research and educational efforts. Continued exploration into microbial landscapes, diagnostic methodologies, and treatment modalities will further refine our understanding of this clinical entity. Through this comprehensive approach, healthcare providers can contribute to improved patient outcomes, enhanced diagnostic precision, and the effective management of this intriguing facet of sinus pathology.

References

Abreu, N. A., Nagalingam, N. A., Song, Y., Roediger, F. C., Pletcher, S. D., Goldberg, A. N., and Lynch, S. V. (2012). Sinus microbiome diversity depletion and Corynebacterium tuberculostearicum enrichment mediates rhinosinusitis. *Science translational medicine*, 4(151), 151ra124. https://doi.org/10.1126/scitranslmed.3003783.

Akhondi, H., Woldemariam, B., and Rajasurya, V. Fungal Sinusitis. [Updated 2023 Jul 3]. In: *StatPearls* [Internet]. Treasure Island (FL): StatPearls Publishing; 2023 Jan-. Available from: https://www.ncbi.nlm.nih.gov/books/NBK551496/.

Al-Mujaini, A., Wali, U., and Alkhabori, M. (2009). Functional endoscopic sinus surgery: indications and complications in the ophthalmic field. *Oman medical journal*, 24(2), 70–80. https://doi.org/10.5001/omj.2009.18.

Al-Saadi, M. A., and Sultan, S. S. N. (2018). Effect of Ceftriaxone versus Amoxicillin + Clavulanic Acid for Treatment of Acute Bacterial Rhino Sinusitis: Short Course Therapy. *Open access Macedonian journal of medical sciences*, 6(8), 1419–1422. https://doi.org/10.3889/oamjms.2018.329.

Areizaga-Madina, M., Pardal-Peláez, B., and Montero, J. (2023). Microbiology of Maxillary Sinus Infections: Systematic Review on the Relationship of Infectious Sinus Pathology with Oral Pathology. *Oral*, 3(1), 134–145. MDPI AG. Retrieved from http://dx.doi.org/10.3390/oral3010012.

Badiee, P., Gandomi, B., Sabz, G., Khodami, B., Choopanizadeh, M., and Jafarian, H. (2015). Evaluation of nested PCR in diagnosis of fungal rhinosinusitis. *Iranian journal of microbiology*, 7(1), 62–66.

Bandres, M. V., Modi, P., and Sharma, S. Aspergillus Fumigatus. [Updated 2023 Aug 8]. In: *StatPearls* [Internet]. Treasure Island (FL): StatPearls Publishing; 2023 Jan-. Available from: https://www.ncbi.nlm.nih.gov/books/ NBK482464/.

Bell, G. W., Joshi, B. B., and Macleod, R. I. (2011). Maxillary sinus disease: diagnosis and treatment. *British dental journal*, 210(3), 113–118. https://doi.org/10.1038/sj.bdj.2011.47.

Boncristiani, H. F., Criado, M. F., and Arruda, E. (2009). Respiratory Viruses. *Encyclopedia of Microbiology*, 500–518. https://doi.org/10.1016/B978-012373944-5.00314-X.

Bromberg, N., and Brizuela, M., Dental Cone Beam Computed Tomography. [Updated 2023 Apr 19]. In: *StatPearls* [Internet]. Treasure Island (FL): StatPearls Publishing; 2023 Jan-. Available from: https://www.ncbi.nlm.nih.gov/books/NBK592390/.

Brook, I. (2005). Microbiology of acute and chronic maxillary sinusitis associated with an odontogenic origin. *The Laryngoscope*, 115(5), 823–825. https://doi.org/10.1097/01.MLG.0000157332.17291.FC.

Craig, J. R., Poetker, D. M., Aksoy, U., Allevi, F., et al. (2021). Diagnosing odontogenic sinusitis: An international multidisciplinary consensus statement. *International forum of allergy & rhinology*, 11(8), 1235–1248. https://doi.org/10.1002/alr.22777.

Davis, W. E., Templer, J., and Parsons, D. S. (1996). Anatomy of the paranasal sinuses. *Otolaryngologic clinics of North America*, 29(1), 57–74.

DeBoer, D. L., and Kwon, E. Acute Sinusitis. [Updated 2023 Aug 7]. In: *StatPearls* [Internet]. Treasure Island (FL): StatPearls Publishing; 2023 Jan-. Available from: https://www.ncbi.nlm.nih.gov/books/NBK547701/.

Fastenberg, J. H., Hsueh, W. D., Mustafa, A., Akbar, N. A., and Abuzeid, W. M. (2016). Biofilms in chronic rhinosinusitis: Pathophysiology and therapeutic strategies. *World journal of otorhinolaryngology - head and neck surgery*, 2(4), 219–229. https://doi.org/10.1016/j.wjorl.2016.03.002.

Gosau, M., Rink, D., Driemel, O., and Draenert, F. G. (2009). Maxillary sinus anatomy: a cadaveric study with clinical implications. *Anatomical record (Hoboken, N.J. : 2007)*, 292(3), 352–354. https://doi.org/10.1002/ar.20859.

Hauman, C. H., Chandler, N. P., and Tong, D. C. (2002). Endodontic implications of the maxillary sinus: a review. *International endodontic journal*, 35(2), 127–141. https://doi.org/10.1046/j.0143-2885.2001.00524.x.

Iwanaga, J., Wilson, C., Lachkar, S., Tomaszewski, K. A., Walocha, J. A., and Tubbs, R. S. (2019). Clinical anatomy of the maxillary sinus: application to sinus floor augmentation. *Anatomy & cell biology*, 52(1), 17–24. https://doi.org/10.5115/acb.2019.52.1.17.

Jacobs, S. E., Lamson, D. M., St George, K., and Walsh, T. J. (2013). Human rhinoviruses. *Clinical microbiology reviews*, 26(1), 135–162. https://doi.org/10.1128/CMR.00077-12.

Kim, S. M. (2019). Definition and management of odontogenic maxillary sinusitis. *Maxillofacial plastic and reconstructive surgery*, 41(1), 13. https://doi.org/10.1186/s40902-019-0196-2.

Lee, K. C., and Lee, S. J. (2010). Clinical features and treatments of odontogenic sinusitis. *Yonsei medical journal*, 51(6), 932–937. https://doi.org/10.3349/ymj.2010.51.6.932.

Little, R. E., Long, C. M., Loehrl, T. A., and Poetker, D. M. (2018). Odontogenic sinusitis: A review of the current literature. *Laryngoscope investigative otolaryngology*, 3(2), 110–114. https://doi.org/10.1002/lio2.147.

Mahdavinia, M., Keshavarzian, A., Tobin, M. C., Landay, A. L., and Schleimer, R. P. (2016). A comprehensive review of the nasal microbiome in chronic rhinosinusitis (CRS). *Clinical and experimental allergy: journal of the British Society for Allergy and Clinical Immunology*, 46(1), 21–41. https://doi.org/10.1111/cea.12666.

Mehra, P., and Jeong, D. (2009). Maxillary sinusitis of odontogenic origin. *Current allergy and asthma reports*, 9(3), 238–243. https://doi.org/10.1007/s11882-009-0035-0.

Peral-Cagigal, B., Redondo-González, L. M., and Verrier-Hernández, A. (2014). Invasive maxillary sinus aspergillosis: A case report successfully treated with voriconazole and surgical debridement. *Journal of clinical and experimental dentistry*, 6(4), e448–e451. https://doi.org/10.4317/jced.51571.

Peñarrocha-Oltra, S., Soto-Peñaloza, D., Bagán-Debón, L., Bagan, J. V., and Peñarrocha-Oltra, D. (2020). Association between maxillary sinus pathology and odontogenic lesions in patients evaluated by cone beam computed tomography. A systematic review and meta-analysis. *Medicina oral, patologia oral y cirugia bucal*, 25(1), e34–e48. https://doi.org/10.4317/medoral.23172.

Psillas, G., Papaioannou, D., Petsali, S., Dimas, G. G., and Constantinidis, J. (2021). Odontogenic maxillary sinusitis: A comprehensive review. *Journal of dental sciences*, 16(1), 474–481. https://doi.org/10.1016/j.jds.2020.08.001.

Puhakka, T., Mäkelä, M. J., Alanen, A., Kallio, T., Korsoff, L., Arstila, P., Leinonen, M., Pulkkinen, M., Suonpää, J., Mertsola, J., and Ruuskanen, O. (1998). Sinusitis in the common cold. *The Journal of allergy and clinical immunology*, 102(3), 403–408. https://doi.org/10.1016/s0091-6749(98)70127-7.

Rujanavej, V., Soudry, E., Banaei, N., Baron, E. J., Hwang, P. H., and Nayak, J. V. (2013). Trends in incidence and susceptibility among methicillin-resistant Staphylococcus aureus isolated from intranasal cultures associated with rhinosinusitis. *American journal of rhinology & allergy*, 27(2), 134–137. https://doi.org/10.2500/ajra.2013.27.3858.

Sawada, S., and Matsubara, S. (2021). Microbiology of Acute Maxillary Sinusitis in Children. *The Laryngoscope*, 131(10), E2705–E2711. https://doi.org/10.1002/lary.29564.

Smith, B., and Johnson, L. (2018). Postoperative care after dental extractions: A guide for patients. *Journal of Oral Surgery*, 25(4), 132-137.

Yoshiura, K., Ban, S., Hijiya, T., Yuasa, K., et al. (1993). Analysis of maxillary sinusitis using computed tomography. *Dento maxillo facial radiology*, 22(2), 86–92. https://doi.org/10.1259/dmfr.22.2.8375560.

Biographical Sketch

Dr. Hema Suryawanshi

Prof (Dr) Hema Suryawanshi currently serves as the Dean and Head of the Department of Oral Pathology and Microbiology at Chhattisgarh Dental College & Research Institute, India. Her expertise lies in Department of Oral Pathology and Microbiology, where she has demonstrated a commitment to both academics and research. As an academician, Dr. Suryawanshi plays a crucial role in shaping the future of dental professionals through her leadership in the oral pathology and microbiology department. Dr. Suryawanshi's research endeavors have resulted in numerous publications in renowned journals, reflecting her dedication to advancing knowledge in the field. Her work contributes to the broader academic and scientific community, enriching our understanding of oral health and pathology.

With a passion for both education and research, Dr. Hema Suryawanshi stands as a notable figure in the dental community, actively shaping the landscape of oral pathology and microbiology in India.

Dr. Santosh R. Patil

Dr. Santosh R. Patil is a proficient Oral Physician and maxillofacial radiologist, currently holding the position of Professor in the Department of Oral Medicine and Radiology at Chhattisgarh Dental College & Research Institute, India. Dr. Patil is a prolific researcher, with numerous articles published in renowned journals, reflecting his dedication to advancing knowledge in the field. His multifaceted contributions and academic leadership mark him as a notable figure in dental education and research.

Chapter 3

The Role of Maxillary Sinus in Dental Infections: A Review of Current Knowledge and Clinical Implications

**Santosh R. Patil[1],*, BDS, MDS, PhD
and Mohmed Isaqali Karobari[2,3], BDS, MScD, *MFDS. RCPS(Galsg)*, PhD Scholar**

[1]Department of Oral Medicine and Radiology, Chhattisgarh Dental College and Research Institute, India
[2] Dental Research Unit, Centre for Global Health Research, Saveetha Institute of Medical and Technical Sciences, Chennai, Tamil Nadu, India
[3]Centre for Dental Health Research, Saveetha Dental Collegeand Hospitals, Saveetha Institute of Medicaland Technical Sciences University,Chennai, Tamil Nadu, India

Abstract

Maxillary sinusitis is a common complication of dental infections, especially those involving the upper molars. It occurs when the infection spreads from the tooth roots to the maxillary sinus, resulting in inflammation of the sinus lining and the accumulation of pus. This condition can cause significant discomfort and pain, and if left untreated, it can lead to serious complications such as the spread of the infection to other parts of the body.

This chapter provides a comprehensive overview of maxillary sinusitis in the context of dental infections. The article covers the anatomy and physiology of the maxillary sinus, the pathophysiology of sinusitis, and the clinical presentation of maxillary sinusitis in dental infections. The article also discusses the diagnosis and management of

---

*Corresponding Author's Email:drpsantosh@gmail.com.

In: Maxillary Sinus Diseases
Editor: Anisha Webb
ISBN: 979-8-89113-534-5
© 2024 Nova Science Publishers, Inc.

this condition, including the use of imaging modalities, antibiotics, and surgical intervention.

Furthermore, the chapter highlights the importance of early diagnosis and management of maxillary sinusitis to prevent complications and improve patient outcomes. The chapter concludes with a discussion of future directions for research in this area, including the need for more robust evidence to guide clinical decision-making and the potential role of novel therapies such as probiotics in the management of maxillary sinusitis in dental infections.

Keywords: maxillary sinus, dental infections, dental pathology, sinusitis, odontogenic infection

Introduction

The maxillary sinus, also known as the antrum of Highmore, is the largest of the paranasal sinuses and is situated in close proximity to the upper posterior teeth. This unique anatomical relationship with the oral cavity gives rise to significant clinical implications, as dental infections can extend into the maxillary sinus, leading to a spectrum of challenges for both dental and medical practitioners. To effectively address these issues, it is crucial to comprehend the role of the maxillary sinus in dental infections (Iwanaga, Joe et al., 2019). This chapter aims to provide a comprehensive exploration of this intricate relationship by delving into the anatomical and physiological aspects of the maxillary sinus, its interactions with adjacent dental structures, the potential pathways of infection, diagnostic approaches, available treatment modalities, and the paramount importance of interdisciplinary collaboration in managing these complex clinical scenarios.

The maxillary sinus plays a pivotal role in maintaining overall oral and sinus health, and its association with dental structures is integral to understanding the nature of odontogenic infections that involve this anatomical cavity (White et al., 2019). Dental practitioners frequently encounter patients presenting with sinus-related complaints that may originate from dental issues. Accurate diagnosis and timely management are essential to alleviate patient suffering and prevent complications. Therefore, a thorough understanding of the relationship between dental structures and the maxillary sinus is fundamental for clinicians.

This chapter will provide a detailed exploration of the maxillary sinus's anatomy, focusing on its proximity to the dental structures, and the mechanisms by which dental infections can extend into the sinus. The various clinical presentations of these infections will be discussed, shedding light on the common symptoms and signs that may manifest in affected patients. Subsequently, the diagnostic approaches for identifying maxillary sinus infections of dental origin will be outlined, emphasizing the importance of clinical, radiographic, and sometimes microbiological assessments.

The management of maxillary sinus infections of dental origin constitutes a multi-faceted approach, involving systemic antibiotics, dental interventions, and, in some cases, sinus procedures. The choice of treatment depends on the severity of the infection, the presence of complications, and the patient's overall health. This chapter will provide a comprehensive overview of the treatment options available, detailing the roles of antibiotics, dental procedures, and sinus surgeries.

Recognizing the clinical implications of maxillary sinus infections of dental origin is imperative. These infections can present with a variety of symptoms that may mimic other sinus conditions, making their accurate diagnosis and differentiation crucial. Moreover, these cases often require a collaborative effort between dental and medical professionals. The importance of an interdisciplinary approach in managing these infections will be highlighted, as it allows for a more comprehensive evaluation and ensures the well-being of the patient.

Furthermore, prevention and patient education are key aspects of managing maxillary sinus infections of dental origin. Preventive dentistry is essential in averting the development of dental infections that may extend into the maxillary sinus. Regular dental check-ups, prompt treatment of dental caries, and periodontal diseases can significantly reduce the risk of complications. Additionally, educating patients about the signs and symptoms of dental infections that may involve the maxillary sinus is crucial. Early recognition of these symptoms can lead to timely intervention, reducing the risk of complications and improving patient outcomes.

Anatomy and Physiology of the Maxillary Sinus

Anatomy of the Maxillary Sinus

The maxillary sinus, also known as the antrum of Highmore, is a paired pyramidal-shaped cavity located within the maxillary bone. It is situated in the facial skeleton, superior to the oral cavity, and inferior to the orbit. Here, we will elaborate on the anatomy of the maxillary sinus in a more descriptive manner:

Location: The maxillary sinus is located within the maxillary bone, one on each side of the face. It occupies a significant portion of the mid-face region, with its base extending into the alveolar process of the maxilla.

Shape and Size: The maxillary sinus exhibits a pyramidal or pyramid-like shape, with its apex pointing upward and its base extending into the maxillary bone. The size of the maxillary sinus can vary among individuals, and it may also differ between the right and left sides of the face (Gosau, M et al., 2009).

Boundaries:

- The superior boundary of the maxillary sinus is formed by the floor of the orbit, which separates it from the eye socket.
- Posteriorly, the maxillary sinus is bounded by the pterygopalatine fossa, a space located deep in the mid-face.
- The inferior boundary is defined by the alveolar process of the maxilla, which contains the roots of the maxillary posterior teeth.
- The medial wall of the maxillary sinus is closely related to the nasal cavity. These two structures are separated by a thin bony partition called the semilunar hiatus. This hiatus contains a small opening that allows for communication between the maxillary sinus and the nasal cavity. The size and precise location of the semilunar hiatus can vary among individuals.

Relationship with Teeth: The roots of the maxillary posterior teeth, including the first and second molars, are often situated in close proximity to the floor of the maxillary sinus. In some cases, the dental roots may even project into the sinus cavity. Anatomical variations in the position and angulation of dental roots can significantly impact the relationship between teeth and the maxillary sinus.

Function: The primary function of the maxillary sinus is twofold. Firstly, it serves to reduce the weight of the skull, which contributes to making the head more manageable. Secondly, it plays a role in enhancing the resonance of the voice. Additionally, the maxillary sinus is part of the respiratory system. It helps filter, humidify, and warm inspired air before it enters the lower respiratory tract. The sinus contains a mucous membrane lining that produces mucus to trap and eliminate foreign particles from the inspired air.

Blood Supply and Innervation: Blood supply to the maxillary sinus is provided by branches of the maxillary artery, which is a major branch of the external carotid artery. Innervation to the maxillary sinus is carried out by the maxillary division of the trigeminal nerve, specifically the maxillary nerve (V2).

Development: The maxillary sinus starts to develop during early childhood and continues to grow and enlarge throughout an individual's lifetime. The rate and extent of this growth can vary among people. This developmental aspect is crucial because it can influence the proximity of dental structures to the maxillary sinus. An understanding of this growth is vital for both medical and dental procedures, especially in cases where dental conditions may extend into the sinus (Gosau, M et al., 2009).

Physiology of the Maxillary Sinus

The maxillary sinus, one of the paranasal sinuses, is an air-filled cavity located within the maxillary bone, which forms the upper jaw. It serves a range of physiological functions that contribute to the overall health and well-being of the respiratory and craniofacial systems.

Facial Skeleton Lightening: One of the primary functions of the maxillary sinus is to reduce the weight of the facial skeleton. The human skull consists of various bones, and the maxillary sinus is strategically positioned within the maxillary bone. By containing air instead of solid bone, it significantly decreases the overall weight of the facial skeleton. This lightening effect is particularly advantageous, as it allows for more efficient chewing and speaking, reduces the strain on facial muscles, and facilitates the overall balance of the facial structure.

Respiratory Air Conditioning: The maxillary sinus plays a vital role in conditioning the air we breathe. It helps to humidify and warm inspired air before it reaches the lower respiratory passages. The respiratory epithelium that lines the sinus secretes mucus, which serves to humidify the incoming air. The warming of air is essential to prevent thermal shock to the lower respiratory tract when inhaling cold air, particularly in cold environments. The air conditioning function helps to maintain the optimal temperature and humidity for the delicate structures of the respiratory system (Sieron, H L et al., 2020).

Mucociliary Clearance: The respiratory epithelium in the maxillary sinus generates mucus to trap particulate matter, such as dust, bacteria, and other foreign particles, that are present in the inhaled air. The mucus contains various defense mechanisms, including antibodies and antimicrobial proteins, which help in protecting the respiratory system from infections and irritants. The cilia, tiny hair-like structures present on the surface of the respiratory epithelium, continuously beat in coordinated motions to move the mucus layer and trapped particles towards the natural drainage pathways. This ensures that the sinus remains clear of foreign debris and maintains its normal physiological functioning.

Ostium and Mucus Drainage: To maintain sinus health and proper physiological functioning, the mucus produced in the maxillary sinus must be continually cleared. This is achieved through the ostium, a small opening that connects the maxillary sinus to the nasal cavity. The ostium allows for the natural flow of mucus, carrying any trapped particles and secretions from the sinus, into the nasal cavity. Once in the nasal cavity, the mucus can be further cleared through the process of swallowing or expectoration. This drainage mechanism is crucial for preventing the accumulation of mucus and preventing infections within the maxillary sinus (Chanavaz, M 1990).

Relationship Between Maxillary Sinus and Adjacent Dental Structures

Proximity to Upper Posterior Teeth

The most significant relationship between the maxillary sinus and dental structures exists in the vicinity of the upper posterior teeth, specifically the maxillary molars and premolars (6). The roots of these teeth are often in close proximity to the floor of the maxillary sinus, with some even projecting into the sinus itself (Fry, Ramesh Ram et al., 2016). This close anatomical relationship creates the potential for dental infections to extend into the sinus and vice versa.

Maxillary Sinus Floor and Alveolar Ridge

The floor of the maxillary sinus and the alveolar ridge, where the roots of the maxillary teeth are anchored, are separated by a thin layer of cortical bone. This bone is sometimes referred to as the alveolar process and may be as thin as 0.5 to 1 mm in certain areas (8). The proximity of the roots to the sinus floor and the variable thickness of this bone are crucial factors in the dynamics of dental infections involving the maxillary sinus (Kilic, Cenk et al., 2010).

Periapical Lesions and Dental Pathology

Periapical lesions, which often result from untreated dental caries or periodontal diseases, can lead to bone resorption at the apices of teeth. If these lesions involve the maxillary posterior teeth, they can create a communication pathway between the oral cavity and the maxillary sinus, allowing for the spread of infection. Such communication can occur through the root apices or lateral accessory canals (Nunes, Carla A B C M et al., 2016).

Pathways of Infection from Dental Structures to the Maxillary Sinus

Dental infections involving the maxillary sinus typically follow several pathways. These pathways can be categorized into direct and indirect routes, each with its own clinical implications (Mehra et al., 2009).

Direct Pathways

Direct pathways involve the direct extension of infection from dental structures into the maxillary sinus. These pathways are often associated with periapical lesions and occur when infections spread through:

- Apical Foramen: Infections originating within the dental pulp can extend through the apical foramen of the tooth's root and gain access to the surrounding bone. From there, they can breach the cortical bone separating the dental apex from the sinus floor.
- Perforations: Iatrogenic factors, such as overzealous dental procedures or accidental perforations, can create direct openings between the oral cavity and the maxillary sinus. This can allow bacteria to directly invade the sinus.

Indirect Pathways

Indirect pathways involve the transmission of infection from dental structures to the maxillary sinus through intermediary structures or spaces. These pathways often include:

- Periodontal Ligament: Infections of periodontal origin can travel along the periodontal ligament and penetrate the thin alveolar bone, eventually reaching the sinus floor (12).
- Lateral Accessory Canals: Dental roots may have lateral accessory canals that can serve as pathways for infection. These accessory canals can allow bacteria to escape from the pulp chamber and invade the surrounding bone, potentially reaching the sinus (13).
- Schneiderian Membrane Perforation: The Schneiderian membrane, which lines the maxillary sinus, is a mucous membrane that can be inadvertently perforated during dental procedures. Such perforations can create a route for infection to enter the sinus (14).

ClinicalPresentation of Maxillary Sinus Infections of Dental Origin

Dental infections that extend into the maxillary sinus can present with a variety of clinical symptoms. These symptoms are often non-specific and may overlap with other conditions affecting the maxillary sinus (Pokorny et al., 2013). Clinicians need to consider the possibility of dental involvement when evaluating patients with the following complaints:

Facial Pain and Tenderness

Patients with dental infections involving the maxillary sinus may experience pain and tenderness over the affected area. The pain is typically localized to the region of the infected tooth and may radiate to the cheek and infraorbital area. It is often aggravated by mastication or changes in head position (Mehra et al., 2004).

Purulent Nasal Discharge

Dental infections that communicate with the maxillary sinus can lead to the presence of purulent nasal discharge, also known as rhinorrhea. The discharge may be intermittent and may have a foul odor. Clinicians should differentiate this from other causes of rhinorrhea, such as rhinosinusitis (Mehra et al., 2004).

Maxillary Toothache

Patients may complain of persistent or recurrent toothache in the upper posterior teeth. The pain may be triggered by hot or cold stimuli and can be exacerbated by lying down, as sinus congestion can increase pressure on the affected tooth (Psillas et al., 2021).

Sinus Congestion and Headache

Maxillary sinus infections of dental origin can lead to sinus congestion, often associated with a dull, aching headache. Patients may also experience nasal stuffiness and a sense of fullness in the affected side of the face (Taschieri, Silvio et al., 2017).

Swelling and Tenderness of the Buccal and Palatal Tissues

In advanced cases, swelling and tenderness of the buccal and palatal soft tissues may be observed. This is often due to the spread of infection into the surrounding soft tissues, resulting in cellulitis (Taschieri, Silvio et al., 2017).

Diagnosis of Maxillary Sinus Infections of Dental Origin

The diagnosis of maxillary sinus infections with dental origins can be challenging due to the non-specific clinical presentation and the potential overlap of symptoms with other sinus conditions. A combination of clinical, radiographic, and sometimes microbiological assessments is essential for an accurate diagnosis (Simuntis, Regimantas et al., 2014).

Clinical Examination

A thorough clinical examination should include:

- Intraoral Examination: Evaluation of the affected teeth, periodontal tissues, and soft tissue integrity. The clinician should check for signs of swelling, redness, and tenderness.
- Extraoral Examination: Assessment of facial asymmetry, palpation of the maxillary sinus area, and identification of any swelling or tenderness (Kim, Soung Min., 2019).

Radiographic Evaluation

Radiographic imaging is crucial for diagnosing and assessing dental infections involving the maxillary sinus. The following radiographic modalities are commonly employed:

- Periapical Radiography: Periapical radiographs are useful for visualizing the apical areas of the teeth, detecting periapical lesions, and assessing the proximity of dental roots to the sinus floor.
- Panoramic Radiography: Panoramic radiographs provide a comprehensive view of the maxillary arch and are valuable for evaluating the overall dental and sinus anatomy (Bisla, Suman et al., 2022).
- Cone Beam Computed Tomography (CBCT): CBCT offers three-dimensional imaging of the maxillary sinus and its relationship with dental structures. It is particularly helpful in identifying the extent of infection and the presence of anatomical variations (Cymerman, Jerome J. et al., 2011).

Microbiological Assessment
When clinical and radiographic findings are inconclusive, microbiological assessment may be necessary. This involves taking a sample of any purulent

discharge or tissue for culture and sensitivity testing. Identifying the specific causative organisms can guide antibiotic therapy (Brook, Itzhak., 2006).

Treatment Options for Maxillary Sinus Infections of Dental Origin

The management of maxillary sinus infections with dental origins necessitates a multi-faceted approach. The choice of treatment depends on the severity of the infection, the presence of complications, and the patient's overall health (Aukštakalnis, Rokas et al., 2018; Starkey et al., 2019).

Antibiotics

Systemic antibiotics are often prescribed to control the infection in conjunction with dental treatments. The choice of antibiotics should be guided by the results of microbiological testing whenever possible. Commonly used antibiotics include amoxicillin/clavulanic acid, clindamycin, and metronidazole.

Dental Interventions

Dental interventions are the cornerstone of managing these infections. The appropriate dental procedures may include:

- Root Canal Therapy: When periapical lesions are identified as the source of infection, root canal therapy is often performed to remove necrotic tissue and seal the root canals to prevent reinfection.
- Tooth Extraction: In cases where the affected tooth is non-restorable or has a poor prognosis, extraction may be necessary.
- Surgical Removal of Infected Tissue: In cases with significant bone loss or abscess formation, surgical debridement may be required to remove infected tissue.

Sinus Procedures

In some instances, particularly when complications arise, sinus procedures may be necessary:

- Caldwell-Luc Procedure: The Caldwell-Luc procedure is a surgical technique that provides access to the maxillary sinus through the canine fossa. It is often used to remove dental foreign bodies or to address chronic sinusitis related to dental infections (Kende, Prajwalit et al., 2019).
- Endoscopic Sinus Surgery: Endoscopic sinus surgery is a minimally invasive approach that can be used to address complications, such as sinusitis or mucoceles, associated with dental infections (Kende, Prajwalit et al., 2019).

Symptomatic Relief

Patients may require symptomatic relief for pain and congestion. Analgesics and decongestants can be recommended to alleviate discomfort and improve nasal breathing.

Clinical Implications and Interdisciplinary Approach

Understanding the relationship between dental structures and the maxillary sinus is vital for both dental and medical practitioners. There are several clinical implications and the importance of an interdisciplinary approach in managing maxillary sinus infections of dental origin (Mehra et al., 2004).

Differential Diagnosis

Clinicians should be aware of the possibility of dental infections extending into the maxillary sinus when evaluating patients with sinus-related complaints. Accurate diagnosis and appropriate referral are critical for effective treatment.

Multidisciplinary Collaboration

Management of maxillary sinus infections of dental origin often requires collaboration between dental and medical professionals. Dentists and oral surgeons work in conjunction with otolaryngologists and maxillofacial surgeons to provide comprehensive care (Mehra et al., 2004).

Prevention

Preventive dentistry is essential in averting the development of dental infections that may extend into the maxillary sinus. Regular dental check-ups, prompt treatment of dental caries, and periodontal diseases can reduce the risk of complications.

Patient Education

Educating patients about the signs and symptoms of dental infections that may involve the maxillary sinus is essential. Early recognition of these symptoms can lead to timely intervention, reducing the risk of complications.

Conclusion

The maxillary sinus is a critical anatomical structure with a unique relationship to adjacent dental structures. Understanding the role of the maxillary sinus in dental infections is paramount for dental and medical professionals. This chapter has explored the anatomy and physiology of the maxillary sinus, its relationship with dental structures, pathways of infection, clinical presentation, diagnostic methods, and treatment options. It has also emphasized the importance of a multidisciplinary approach to managing these infections.

By recognizing the intricate interplay between dental and maxillary sinus health, clinicians can provide timely and effective care, improving patient outcomes and quality of life. Continuing research in this field will further enhance our understanding of the role of the maxillary sinus in dental infections and contribute to more efficient diagnostic and treatment strategies.

Disclaimer

None.

References

Archer, R. K., Harlan, W., &Verbic, J. (2002). Dental Infections as a Source of Sinus Disease. *Otolaryngology-Head and Neck Surgery*, 127(4), 387-389. doi:10.1067/mhn.2002.127034.

Brook, I. (2006). Sinusitis of Odontogenic Origin. *Otolaryngology--Head and Neck Surgery*, 135(3), 349-355. doi:10.1016/j.otohns.2005.10.059.

Chanavaz, M. (1990). Maxillary Sinus: Anatomy, Physiology, Surgery, and Bone Grafting Related to Implantology--Eleven Years of Surgical Experience (1979-1990). *The Journal of Oral Implantology*, 16(3), 199-209.

Cymerman, J. J., Cymerman, J. A., &Kratochvil, F. J. (2009). Odontogenic sinusitis: a review of the current literature. *The Laryngoscope*, 119(6), 1109-1113. doi:10.1002/lary.20284.

Fry, R. R., Patidar, R. M., &Gopalkrishnan, K. (2016). Proximity of maxillary posterior teeth roots to maxillary sinus and adjacent structures using Denta scan®. *Indian Journal of Dentistry*, 7(3), 126-130. doi:10.4103/0975-962X.189339.

Gosau, M., Rink, D., Draenert, F. G., &Ettl, T. (2013). Odontogenic sinusitis: a review of the current literature. *Clinical Oral Investigations*, 17(1), 59-64. doi:10.1007/s00784-011-0614-3.

Iwanaga, J., Watanabe, K., Bobek, S. L., et al. (2019). Clinical anatomy of the maxillary sinus: application to sinus floor augmentation. *Anatomy & Cell Biology*, 52(1), 17-24. doi:10.5115/acb.2019.52.1.17.

Kende, P., Sharma, K., & Chandra, P. (2019). Combined endoscopic and intra-oral approach for chronic maxillary sinusitis of dental origin-a prospective clinical study. *Oral and Maxillofacial Surgery*, 23(4), 429-437. doi:10.1007/s10006-019-00792-z.

Kilic, C., Kamburoğlu, K., Ozen, T., &Balcioglu, H. A. (2010). An Assessment of the Relationship between the Maxillary Sinus Floor and the Maxillary Posterior Teeth Root Tips Using Dental Cone-beam Computerized Tomography. *European Journal of Dentistry*, 4(4), 462-467.

Kim, S. M. (2019). Definition and management of odontogenic maxillary sinusitis. *Maxillofacial Plastic and Reconstructive Surgery*, 41(1), 13. doi:10.1186/s40902-019-0196-2.

Mehra, P., & Jeong, D. (2009). Maxillary sinusitis of odontogenic origin. *Current Allergy and Asthma Reports*, 9(3), 238-243. doi:10.1007/s11882-009-0035-0.

Mehra, P., & Murad, H. (2004). Maxillary sinus disease of odontogenic origin. *Otolaryngologic Clinics of North America*, 37(2), 347-364. doi:10.1016/S0030-6665(03)00171-3.

Nunes, C. A. B. C. M., Guedes, O. A., Almeida, S. M. M., &Ambrosano, G. M. B. (2016). Evaluation of periapical lesions and their association with maxillary sinus abnormalities on cone-beam computed tomographic images. *Journal of Endodontics*, 42(1), 42-46. doi:10.1016/j.joen.2015.09.014.

Pokorny, A., &Tataryn, R. (2013). Clinical and radiologic findings in a case series of maxillary sinusitis of dental origin. *International Forum of Allergy & Rhinology*, 3(12), 973-979. doi:10.1002/alr.21212.

Psillas, G., Samara, M., &Koumoura, F. (2021). Odontogenic maxillary sinusitis: A comprehensive review. *Journal of Dental Sciences*, 16(1), 474-481. doi:10.1016/j.jds.2020.08.001.

Sieron, H. L., Kende, P., & Garagiola, U. (2020). Funktionund Physiologie der Kieferhöhle [Function and physiology of the maxillary sinus]. *HNO*, 68(8), 566-572. doi:10.1007/s00106-020-00869-2.

Simuntis, R., Gervickas, A., &Peciuliene, V. (2014). Odontogenic maxillary sinusitis: a review. *Stomatologija*, 16(2), 39-43.

Starkey, J. L., &Mortman, R. E. (2019). Treatment of Maxillary Sinusitis of Odontogenic Origin: A Case Series. *Compendium of Continuing Education in Dentistry*, 40(8), 516-522.

Taschieri, S., Tsesis, I., Del Fabbro, M., & Rosen, E. (2017). Pathophysiology of sinusitis of odontogenic origin. *Journal of Investigative and Clinical Dentistry*, 8(2). doi:10.1111/jicd.12202.

Whyte, A., &Boeddinghaus, R. (2019). The maxillary sinus: physiology, development, and imaging anatomy. *Dento Maxillo Facial Radiology*, 48(8), 20190205. doi:10.1259/dmfr.20190205.

Chapter 4

Maxillary Sinus Hypoplasia

Mohammad Hatamleh
Zain Al-Qudah
Mohammad Khraisat
Ra'ed Al-ashqar
and Mohannad Al-Qudah[*]

Division of Otolaryngology, Department of Special Surgery, Jordan University of Science and Technology, Irbid, Jordan

Abstract

The maxillary sinus, the largest paranasal sinus, is located below the orbit between the nasal and oral cavities. It begins to develop after the 10th week of gestation, and the cavity becomes identifiable at 16 weeks of gestation age. At birth, the volume of the maxillary sinus is 6–8 mm.It increases with the growth of the nasal cavity, the infraorbital wall, the alveolar process, and the zygomatic process. The final pneumatization of the maxillary sinus occurs principally in a caudal direction after the eruption of the maxillary teeth. The adult size is reached at the age of 15–18-year-old.

Maxillary sinus hypoplasia (MSH) is a relatively uncommon condition. Otolaryngologist, dentist and maxillofacial surgeon aren't usually familiar with this medical term. MSH can be congenital or acquired. It has different classifications and limitation degree of pnumatization. It is usually associated also with abnormalities of the ostiomeatal complex and sinonasal region.The diagnosis is proved by the

---

[*] Corresponding Author: Mohannad Al-Qudah, MD, FACS, FAAOHNS, Professor of Otolaryngology, Department of Special Surgery, Jordan University of Science & Technology, P.O. Box:3030, Irbid (22110), Jordan; Email: malqudah@gmail.com.

In: Maxillary Sinus Diseases
Editor: Anisha Webb
ISBN: 979-8-89113-534-5
© 2024 Nova Science Publishers, Inc.

presence of remarkable radiographic signs on computer tomography. Most cases of MSH do not cause any symptoms. However, proper identification of this clinical entity is fundamental in certain conditions and required medical and surgical management approach modifications to avoid the potential of serious complications.

Keywords: hypoplasia, maxillary sinus, orbit, endoscop, sinusitis, classification, ethmoid

Introduction

Maxillary Sinus Hypoplasia (MSH) is a persistent decrease in maxillary sinus (MS) volume due to a centripetal retraction of the maxillary sinus walls. It occurs when the affecting lower margin of the maxillary sinus doesn't exceed the nasal floor. The involution of the MS walls leads to a relative increase in orbital volume and may result in enopthalmus and hypoglobus [1,2].

MSH has been described as early as 1912. Montgomery in 1964 reported two cases of maxillarysinus mucocele and enopthalmus. These early literature descriptions were restricted to maxillary antrum region with limited consideration to the important adjacent structures in the sinonasal region, namely the ethmoid labyrinth and the orbit [3].

The objective of this chapter is to review the relevant clinical anatomy and embryology of maxillary sinus and to describe the clinical significant of appropriate HMS diagnosis. Various approaches, methods implications and techniques to manage HMS will be discussed along with their advantages and limitations.

Definition and Epidemiology

Karmody et al., in 1977 defined the criteria for MSH based on assessment of the pneumatization of the zygomatic process (lateral extent) and pneumatization of the alveolar process (inferior extent) using plain radiography [4]. Two additional criteria were used by Bassiouny et al., who studied the radiological findings of HMS using four standard plain X-ray views. These criteria included failure of the sinus to develop cephalically toward the orbit leaving the inferior orbital wall in its original curved (concave upward) position, with the infraorbital foramen near the center of the maxilla and diminished expansion of the sinus medially toward the nasal cavity with resulting lateral displacement of the nasal wall [5]. Bolger et al. estimated the volume of the maxillary antrum based on CT software calculations of the area of each image of the hypoplastic sinus in millimeters. They also obtained a "volume estimate ratio" by dividing the volume estimate of the hypoplastic sinus by the volume estimate of the contralateral normal sinus [6].

The advent of functional endoscopic sinus surgery and the wide spread clinical usage of high resolution sinonasal CT scan have led to a better understanding of anatomical variations in this region[2]. The nose and paranasal sinus are considered as one physiological functional unit with a continuous lining mucosa.

In clinical practice, MSH is generally an uncommon condition. Its true incidence is not clear as there are wide variations in reported incidents between different studies. Reported figures range from 1.73 per cent to 10.4 per cent for unilateral and 3.6-7.2 per cent for bilateral MSH in the general adult population [4-7]. There is no significant difference in the incidence based on gender or side of involvement [8]. This variability is contributed mainly to the different methods used for diagnosis MSH and analysis the results. High resolution-three dimensional CT scan and different angled endoscopes allow optimum visualization and detection of detailed tiny changes in the sinonasal region anatomy. On the other hand, old plain radiography and head light mirror rhinoscopy led to misdiagnosis of MSH with maxillary sinusitis, Figure 1.

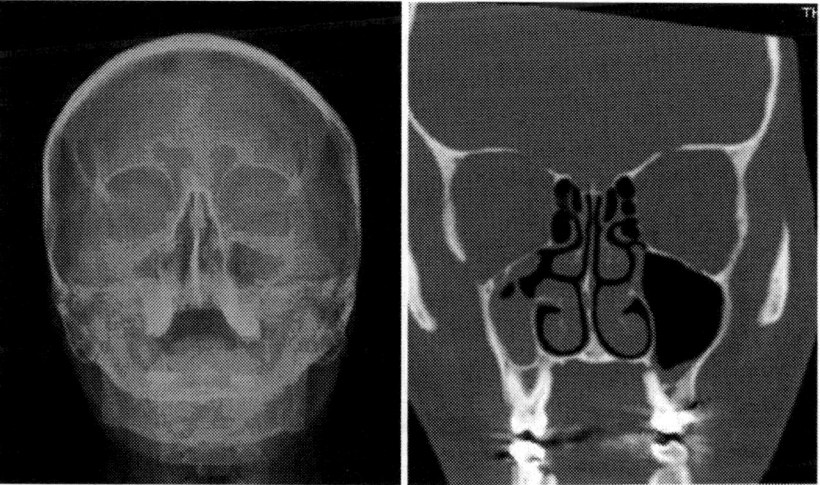

Figure 1. Waters view plain X-ray showing bilateral maxillary opacification with misdiagnosis of right side as normal size maxillary sinus. Coronal CT scan of the same patient revealed type II right sided hypoplastic maxillary sinus.

Clinical Anatomy and Embryology

Description of detailed complex anatomy of the sinonasal region is beyond the scope of this chapter; however, any relevant clinical anatomical and embryological content will be outlined.

The MS is the largest paranasal sinus. It has a pyramidal shape with six walls (posterior, anterior, lateral, medial, and narrow posterior and inferior walls) each wall is formed from a different skull bony part [9, 10].

At birth the maxillary antrum size is about 6-8 mm3. During childhood growth and development, the MS volume expands in several directions toward the inferior orbital wall, nasal cavity, zygomatic process and alveolar process. In the first 8 years of life the MS increases by the rate of 2mm/ year in the vertical and lateral dimensions and by 3 mm per year in the anteroposterior dimension. The lower boundary of the maxillary sinus reaches the level of the nasal cavity floor at the age of 10 years. Subsequent further expansion of MS is primarily achieved in an inferior direction. By late adolescence, the maximum volume of the maxillary sinus is reached while the eruption of the upper teeth is fully completed [8-10].

The floor of the adult sinus usually lies between 5-10 mm below the level of the floor of the nasal cavity. The average sinus size at adulthood measures 33 mm vertically, 23 mm transversely, 34 mm anteroposteriorly, and has a volume of approximately 15 ml [4].

The ethmoid sinuses consist of multiple air cells located within the ethmoid labyrinth of the ethmoid bone and separated by thin bones from the brain and orbit. The ethmoidal labyrinth is divided by multiple obliquely oriented, parallel lamellae. The first lamella is equivalent to the uncinate process of ethmoid bone. This sickle shaped structure projects posteroinferiorly from the ethmoid bone. The ethmoidal infundibulum is a three-dimensional slit-like space bounded by the uncinate process, medially, the orbital lamina of ethmoid bone (lamina papyracea), laterally, and the ethmoidal bulla, posteriorly. The ostiomeal complex is an area located in the middle meatus lateral to the middle turbinate that houses the ostia of the frontal, anterior ethmoid and maxillary sinuses [10, 11].

The outline of the bony orbit is circular with a slightly concave floor at birth. During paranasal sinus pneumatization and facial bone growth, increase in the volume of ethmoid and maxillary sinuses causes extrinsic pressure on the adjacent orbital walls with thinning and flattening of the floor and medial wall of the orbit [5].

The nasal cavity develops from the nasal pits, which are paired depressions on the frontonasal process of the developing embryo. Fusion of various structures in the midline forms the nasal septum that divides the nasal cavity into left and right halves. As the bones of the skull develop around the nasal cavity, air-filled spaces known as paranasal sinuses begin to form within these bones [10].

A close connection is present between the development of the anterior ethmoidal sinuses, the lateral nasal wall and the maxillary sinus. At approximately 6 weeks in utero, evagination of lateral wall mucosa of the olfactory pit forms the principal nasal conchae (superior, middle, and inferior). A second set of mucosal invagination takes place between the middle and inferior conchae in the region of the future middle nasal meatus. This leads to the formation of the secondary conchae. The first and second fuse to form the ethmoidal bulla, and the third (most inferior) forms the uncinate process [9,10].

The ethmoidal infundibulum appears at 10-week gestation age [8]. The ethmoidal sinus bud is formed from the middle meatus at 11 to 12 weeks of gestation. The uncinate process develops at 12 weeks. Thesestructures precede the appearance of the MS bud. The MS develops as a "bud" or "pouch" of the ethmoidal-maxillary recessmucosa at the central part of the middle meatus of the nasal cavity between 14 and 15 weeks of fetal life. Thisevagination penetrates into the maxilla with concurrent resorption of the surrounding bone. At this time, the lateral wall of the nose is already highly developed, and the three turbinates can be seen, consisting of a cartilaginous core with an overlying mucous membrane [9, 10].

At 15 to 16 weeks of gestation, the primitive MS increases in size lateral to the cartilaginous capsule of the nasal cavity before the appearance of the ethmoid bulla at 17 weeks. The primodial posterior ethmoid air cells "bud" independently form from the lateral nasal wall around 18 weeks. Ossification of the anterior maxilla and nasal capsule occurs at 12 weeks, before the primitive MS appears, while the ethmoid sinuses don't ossify until 20-22 weeks [10,11].

Etiology

The exact pathophysiology of HMS has not been identified. Several studies, however, have proposed that chronic negative pressure within the MS resulting from sinus ostial obstruction is the cause [5,6]. Although the specific reason for this antrum ostium blockage is difficult to specify, several mechanisms have been suggested, such as: lateralized middle turbinate or infundibular wall, occlusion secondary to inspissated mucous, mucosal inflammation preventing ostial ventilation, mucocele or nasal polyp compromising ostial ventilation and narrowing of the ostia by infraorbital ethmoid (Haller) air cells [1].

Nasal ventilation is crucial for paranasal sinus pneumatization in similarity to what middle ear ventilation does for temporal bone pneumatization [12]. MS is ventilated physiologically during the expiratory phase of respiration. Normally developed uncinate process is believed to be essential in order to direct the expired air toward the sinus cavity. Abnormal uncinate process, commonly seen in HMS, might also impede mucocilliary clearance of the antrum. These lead to a MS filled with thick secretions rather than air, which retards MS pneumatization and causes hypoplasia [11]. However, it is not clear whether sinusitis is the primary factor or occurs secondary to these anatomical abnormalities.

Hypoplasia of the maxillary sinus can be classified into 3 groups based on the presence of other abnormalities [5]:

1. Isolated hypoplasia, which can be either:

A. primary hypoplasia:(a true embryological failure in the development of the sinus). The MS and uncinate process have a common origin from the cartilaginous nasal capsule and this may explain the high frequency of associated lateral nasal wall structures abnormality seen with MSH patients [11].Tsue et al., reported one case of bilateral MS aplasia and bilateral sinonasal papillamtosis [13]. Human papilloma virus can affect the development of paranasal sinuses by teratogenic effect during intrauterine period.

B. secondary hypoplasia resulting from an arrest of pneumatization caused by sinus infection or sinus trauma (including radiation injury) in childhood. Chewing on one side can induce excessive pressure on one maxilla at different points which leads to a remodeling of the bone as the maxilla slowly adjusts to the stress [5].

2. Hypoplasia associated with regional abnormalities involving the first branchial arch: hypoplasia may be found in disorders such as mandibulofacial dysostosis (Treacher Collins syndrome), craniofacial dysostosis (Crouzon's syndrome), acrocephalosyndactyly (Apert's syndrome), asymmetrical craniostenosis and, occasionally, hare lip and cleft palate.

3. Hypoplasia associated with systemic disorders: in thalassemia the maxilla consists mainly of red bone marrow in an attempt to compensate

erythrocytosis. Fibroprolifrative conditions such as: fibrous dysplasia and Paget'sdisease, as well as inflammatory osteiitis as in Wegener's granulomatosis.

Also, there are many lesions that can cause reduction in the bony sinus lumen:

1) Traumatic: certain surgical procedures, such as Caldwell-Luc procedure and endoscopic sinus surgery as well as healed fractures may lead to bony thickening of the sinus walls and obliteration. The proposed mechanisms include activation of bone formation within the maxilla and the removal of pneumatization canters [7].
2) Inflammatory: chronic sinusitis during the first year of life could cause HMS with sclerosing osteitis.
3) Neoplastic: primary neoplasms and some osteoblastic metastases.

Classification

The most widely accepted and used classification for MSH is that described by Bolger and co-workers in 1990[6]. They used 5- mm coronal CT scans to classify MSH into three types, based on the level of MS pneumatization as well as the shape and development condition of uncincate process. The classification is helpful for preoperative assessment and planning surgical techniques since infundibulotomy is an essential and major step of safe antrostomy.

Type I Bolger's classification is characterized bynormal uncinate process, a well-defined infundibular passage, and mild sinus hypoplasia. Absence or hypoplasia of the uncinate process, an ill-defined infundibular passage, and soft-tissue density opacification of a significantly hypoplastic sinus is considered as Type II, whereas absence of the uncinate process and a profoundly hypoplastic, cleft-like sinus is the Type III.

The majority of HMS cases are type I.Type II accounts for around 30% whereas type III is extremely rare in clinical practice and reported in less than 10% of symptomatic HMS patients [1, 2].

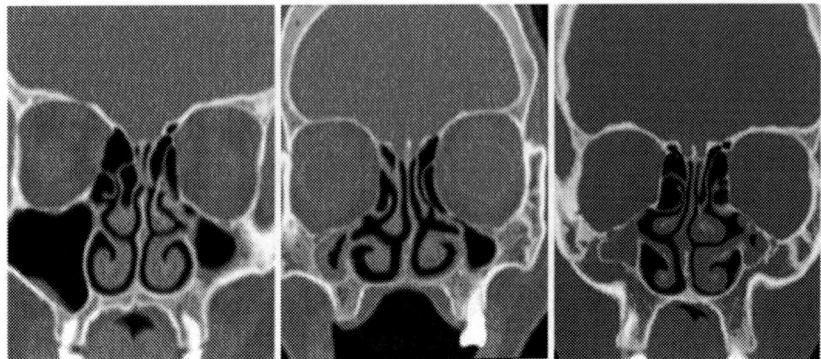

Figure 2. Coronal CT scan of the sinonasal region. Left side picture shows left sided type 1 MSH with well-developed infundibulum. Picture in the middle demonstrates right sided type 2 MSH with abnormally developed uncinate process and narrow infundibulum as a comparison to type 1 MSH in left side. Right sided picture shows type 3 MSH, the sinus appears as cleft like when compared to type 2 MSH on the right side. MSH: Maxillary Sinus Hypoplasia.

Sirikçi et al., recommended inclusion of orbital volume to Bolger type II and III maxillary sinus hypoplasia classification [14]. Mild MSH was considered when the maximum horizontal or vertical diameter of the MS was less than half the maximum orbital diameter on the same side. Severe MSH was considered when both the maximum vertical and horizontal diameters of the maxillary sinus were less than half of the ipsilateral maximum orbital diameter. Orbital volume measurements and comparison with maxillary sinus size can help prevent misdiagnosis of a chronic maxillary sinus atelectasis as a HMS. Awareness of orbital malposition will draw meticulous attention to the surgical limits during uncinate process dissecting which will help in preventing inadvertent serious orbital complications.

Clinical Presentation

The clinical presentation of MSH exhibits considerable variability, encompassing a spectrum. In most patients it's entirely asymptomatic, while other patients may experience different non-specific and non-distinguishable sinonasal symptoms including: rhinorrhea, sneezing, nasal obstruction, headache or chronic sinusitis not responding to conventional therapy [1,2,4,5,6]. MSH classification types may affect the scope of clinical presentation: Type I and type III are less likely to be symptomatic. Type I has a normal drainage pathway therefore no tendency to develop sinusitis or increased risk of orbital penetration in endoscopic surgery, while type III has no sinus airspace to become infected.

Anterior rhinoscopy is usually unremarkable. Endoscopic nasal examination may show anatomical variations in the nasal cavity which are commonly present with HMS such as nasal septal deviation, middle turbinate concha bullosa and maxillary sinus accessory ostium. It usually also shows lateral displacement of the membrane covering the posterior fontanelle, Figure 3 [2, 14].

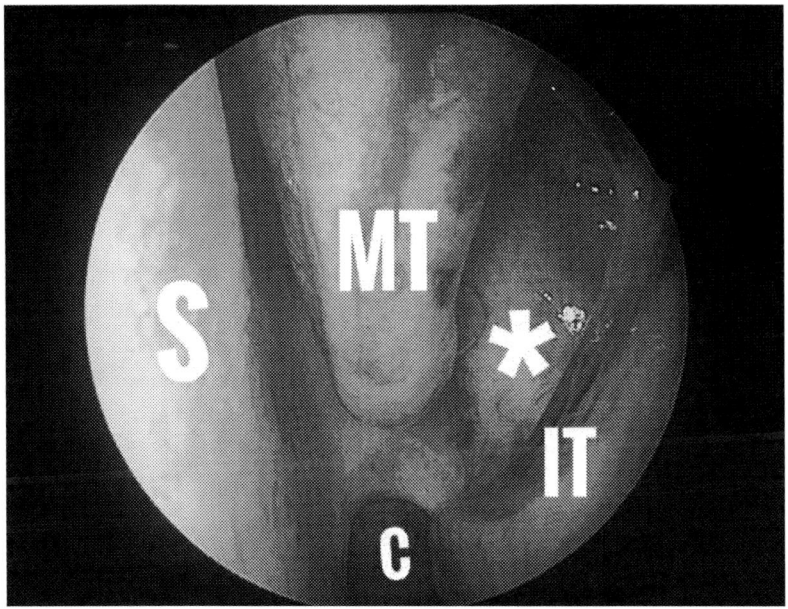

Figure 3. 30 degree rigid nasal endoscopy view of the left nasal cavity demonstrating lateral displacement of maxillary sinus medial wall. S: Septum, MT: Middle Turbinate, IT: Inferior Turbinate, C: Choana, *: Maxillary sinus medial wall.

The two critical ophthalmologic signs are enophthalmos (eye posteriorlydisplaced) and hypoglobus (eye inferiorly displaced).The range of enophthalmos varies from 1 to 6 mm, and the range of hypoglobus varies from 0 to 6 mm. Other common associated ophthalmology signs are upper lidsulcus deepening, eyelid retraction, lid lag and lagophthalmos [1].

Radiographic Characteristics

HMS is best evaluated using computed tomography (CT) scanning. CT scan is superior to other radiological modalities as it shows the ethmoid complex details more clearly, demonstrates the mucoperiosteal lining of the sinuses and provides better visualization of the orbit [7].

CT scans usually show maxillary sinus opacification with a reduction in sinus volume, Figure 2. The posterolateral wall (especially the posterior one-third segment), medial wall and anterior wall of the maxillary sinus may also be found to be concave. Consequently, the orbital size is increased, especially in the vertical dimension. In addition, there is often a collapse and inferior bowing of the orbital floor with widening of the superior and inferior orbital fissures and lateral positioning of the infraorbital neurovascular canal [1,5,6,7,15]. Frequently, the nasal septum is deviated toward the side of the HMS, sometimes associated with a contralateral concha bullosa and ipsilateral elevated canine fossa [2, 14].

Uncinate process may be lateralized against the medial wall of the orbit, hypoplastic or absent. It tends to become fused to the inferomedial orbital wall superiorly, while being demineralized and thinned inferiorly. The infundibulum passage tract may be poorly aerated and obliterated.

Other less common reported CT signs include: enlargement of the pterygopalatine fossa due to a short anteroposterior of the involved maxilla side, and a low lying roof of the ethmoid [14-16].

Differential Diagnosis

The retromaxillary cell should be differentiated from HMS. This cell is an over-expansion of a posterior ethmoidal air cell into the maxillary sinus [14]. It is bounded anteroinferiorly by the junction between the posterior and superior walls of the MS and characterized by drainage into an enlarged superior meatus, reduction in the size of the maxillary sinus and a normal bony orbital cavity [17].

The difference between HMS, chronic maxillary atelectasis and silent sinus syndrome isunclear and confusing [2].Chronic maxillary atelectasis is a descriptive term thatrefers to a persistent decrease in the maxillary sinus volume associated with inward bowing of the sinus walls. It isdiagnosed based on clinical and radiological findings [18]. Kass et al., [19] classified chronic maxillary atelectasis into three stages according to the degree of wall collapse. Instage I, the fontanelle and medial infundibular wall were laterallypositioned. In stage II, one or more osseous walls ofthe maxillary sinus bowed inward. In stage III, markeddeformation of the sinus walls manifested clinically asenophthalmos, hypoglobus and/or midfacial deformity.

The different Bolger classification types of HMS with chronic rhinosinusitis fit within stage II chronicmaxillary atelectasis. Sinonasal symptom severity is inversely related to the chronic maxillary atelectasis stage [2]. Chronic maxillaryatelectasis stages I and II are commonly associated withsinonasal symptoms, whereas stage III is often asymptomaticand presents with orbital deformity [1].

The silent sinus syndrome is an uncommon disorder characterized by painless facial asymmetry, enophthalmos and a spontaneous unilateral maxillary atelectasis with complete or partial opacification of the MS. The clinical characteristics of silent sinus syndrome are almost identical to those of stage III chronic maxillary atelectasis. It appears that stage III chronic maxillary atelectasis may in fact be the final pathway that brings about the asymptomatic spontaneous enophthalmos observed with the entity referred to as silent sinus syndrome [18].

Management

It is important to realize the HMS is an anatomical variant of maxillary sinus that is usually asymptomatic and can be discovered as a coincidental radiological diagnosis. However, its proper recognition is essential before any procedure in the sinonasal region, orbit or oral cavity to avoid serious possible complications such as brain or orbital penetration.

HMS is more prone to medically resistant chronic rhinosinusitis with poor medical response [20]. The condition is usually associated with changes in the ethmoid infundibulum configuration which prevents healthy sinus ventilation and a natural mucociliary drainage pathway [7] Thick, viscid mucopurulent secretions with Methicillin-resistant Staphylococcus aureus is often aspirated from the infected sinus [2].

Functional endoscopic sinus surgery is the best safe and effective surgical procedure for HMS with refractory sinusitis. The classical procedure steps should be tailored to the pre-operative CT scan and intra-operative findings, with the use of additional helpful techniques to avoid potential serious complications [2]. After surgery, the configuration of the maxillary sinus may completely become normal, slightly improve or remain unchanged [2]. Regardless of the final appearance of the sinus after surgery, the evolution of the disease stops with no development of progressive or extensive deformity [21], Figure 4.

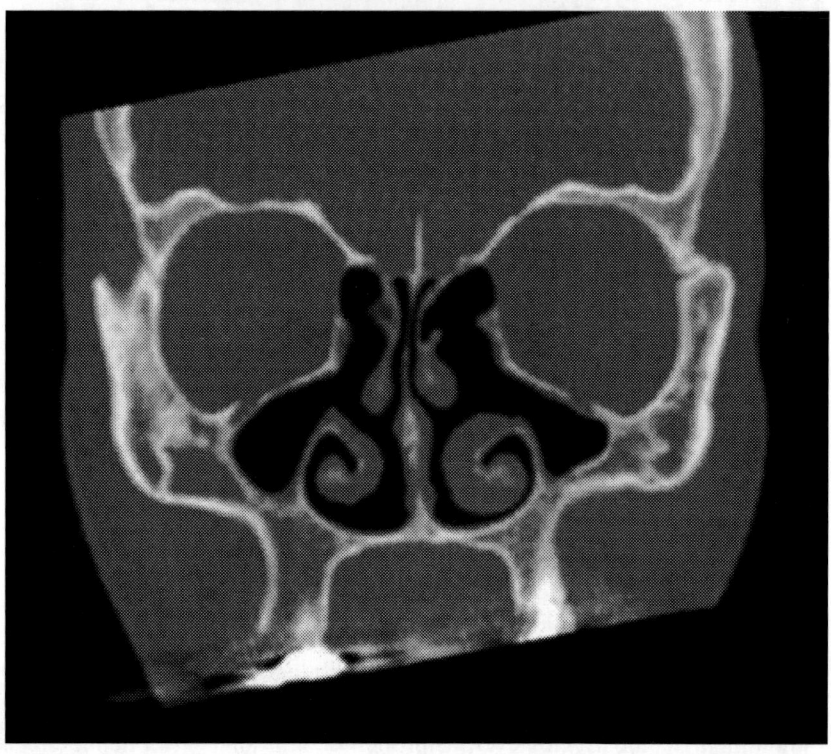

Figure 4. 5- years postoperative coronal CT scan for a patient with bilateral type I MSH demonstrating healthy maxillary sinus mucosa with bilateral patent wide maxillary antrostomy.

Conclusion

MSH is a relatively infrequently faced clinical problem. The clinical presentation may involve non-specific sinonasal symptoms or may be accidentally discovered in radiological images. The etiology is unknown, but likely results from maxillary antrum ostial narrowing compromising normal physiological sinus ventilation. The diagnosis is proved by the presence of remarkable radiographic signs on computer tomography. Symptomatic patients with refractory sinusitis can be managed safely and effectively by endoscopic sinus surgery to establish adequate ventilation through posteriorly positioned antrostomy.

References

[1] Loehrl TA, Hong SH. The hypoplastic maxillary sinus and the orbital floor. *Curr. Opin. Otolaryngol. Head Neck Surg.* (2006) 14(1) :35Y37.
[2] Al-Qudah M, Zubidi A. Functional endoscopic sinus surgery outcome in chronic rhinosinusitis patients with hypoplastic maxillary sinus. *J. Laryngol. Otol.* (2022) 136(5):414-418.
[3] Birkent H, Tosun F, Karahatay S, Akcam T. Progressive maxillary sinus hypoplasia with open ostium. *J. Craniofac. Surg.* (2007) 18(3):706-8.
[4] Karmody CS, Carter B, Vincent ME. Developmental anomalies of the maxillary sinus. *Trans Sect. Otolaryngol. Am. Acad. Ophthalmol. Otolaryngol.* (1977) 84: 723 – 728.
[5] Bassiouny, A., Newlands, W. J., Ali, H., &Zaki, Y. Maxillary sinus hypoplasia and superior orbital fissure asymmetry. *The Laryngoscope* (1982) 92(4), 441–448.
[6] Bolger WE, Woodruff WW Jr, Morehead J, Parsons DS. Maxillary sinus hypoplasia: classification and description of associated uncinate process hypoplasia. *Otolaryngol. Head Neck Surg.* (1990)103(5):759-65.
[7] Salib RJ, Chaudri SA, Rockley TJ. Sinusitis in the hypoplastic maxillary antrum: the crucial role of radiology in diagnosis and management. *J. Laryngol. Otol.* (2001) 115(8):676-8.
[8] Wake, M., Shankar, L., Hawke, M., & Takeno, S. Maxillary sinus hypoplasia, embryology, and radiology. *Archives of otolaryngology--head & neck surgery* (1993) 119(12), 1353–1357.
[9] Whyte A, Boeddinghaus R. The maxillary sinus: physiology, development and imaging anatomy. *Dentomaxillofac. Radiol.* (2019)48(8):20190205.
[10] Neskey D, Eloy JA, Casiano RR. Nasal, septal, and turbinate anatomy and embryology. *Otolaryngol. Clin. North Am.* (2009)42(2):193-205.
[11] Al-Qudah MA. Extra middle turbinate lamellas: a suggested new classification. *Surg. Radiol. Anat.* (2015);37(8):941-5.
[12] Erdem T, Aktas D, Erdem G, Miman MC, Ozturan O. Maxillary sinus hypoplasia. *Rhinology.* (2002) 40(3):150-3.
[13] Tsue TT, Bailet JW, Barlow DW, Makielski KH. Bilateral sinonasalpapillomas in aplastic maxillary sinuses. *Am. J. Otolaryngol.* (1997) 18(4):263-8.
[14] Sirikçi A, Bayazit Y, Gümüsburun E, Bayram M, Kanlikana M. A new approach to the classification of maxillary sinus hypoplasia with relevant clinical implications. *Surg. Radiol. Anat.* (2000)22(5-6):243-7.
[15] Geraghty JJ, Dolan KD. Computed tomography of the hypoplastic maxillary sinus. *Ann. Otol. Rhinol. Laryngol.* (1989)98(11):916-8.

[16] Hanna E, Levine HL, Timen S, Kotton B. Hypoplasia of the Maxillary Antrum: Anatomic Abnormalities, Diagnostic Difficulties and Surgical Implications.*American Journal of Rhinology* (1993)7(3):105-110.

[17] Herzallah IR, Saati FA, Marglani OA, Simsim RF. RetromaxillaryPneumatization of Posterior Ethmoid Air Cells: Novel Description and Surgical Implications. *Otolaryngol. Head Neck Surg.* (2016)155(2):340-6.

[18] Brandt MG, Wright ED. The silent sinus syndrome is a form of chronic maxillary atelectasis: a systematic review of all reported cases. *Am. J. Rhinol.*(2008)22(1):68-73.

[19] Kass ES, Salman S, Rubin PA, Weber AL, Montgomery WW. Chronic maxillary atelectasis. *Ann. Otol. Rhinol.Laryngol.* (1997)106(2):109-16.

[20] Jang YJ, Kim HC, Lee JH, Kim JH. Maxillary sinus hypoplasia with a patent ostiomeatal complex: A therapeutic dilemma. *AurisNasus Larynx.* (2012)39(2):175-9.

[21] Thomas RD, Graham SM, Carter KD, Nerad JA. Management of the orbital floor in silent sinus syndrome. *Am. J. Rhinol.* (2003)17(2):97-100.

Chapter 5

Maxillary Sinusitis of Dental Origin

Mosaad Abdel-Aziz[*], MD
and Ayman S. Megahed, MD

Department of Otolaryngology, Kasr Alainy Faculty of Medicine,
Cairo University, Cairo, Egypt

Abstract

Dental pathology is implicated in causing isolated maxillary sinusitis. The proximity of the roots of upper teeth to the floor of the maxillary sinus could help ascending infection. Failure to identify the offending dental problem can lead to persistent sinus infection and failure of treatment. Odontogenic maxillary sinusitis is usually presented with persistent offensive nasal discharge. Diagnosis of such condition needs dental and otolaryngologic examination. Computed tomography (CT) and/or cone beam computed tomography (CBCT) are important diagnostic tools for patients with odontogenic maxillary sinusitis. Dental causes of maxillary sinusitis are underestimated and may be overlooked by the otolaryngologists, so proper diagnosis is of paramount importance for treatment, as the pathophysiology, microbiology, and treatment differ from those of other types of sinusitis. Sometimes treatment of dental pathology alone is adequate to resolve the condition, however surgical intervention by endoscopic sinus surgery or even Caldwell-Luc operation may be required after treatment of dental problem.

Keywords: maxillary sinusit is, dental infection, odontogenic sinusitis, oroantral fistula

---

[*] Correspondence to: Mosaad Abdel-Aziz, Address: 2 el-salam st., King Faisal, above el-baraka bank, Giza, Cairo, Egypt. Telephone: +201005140161. Fax: +20 225329113. ORCID: 0000-0002-7250-5388. Email: mosabeez@yahoo.com.

In: Maxillary Sinus Diseases
Editor: Anisha Webb
ISBN: 979-8-89113-534-5
© 2024 Nova Science Publishers, Inc.

Introduction

The maxillary sinus is anatomically situated in the mid-face between the eye ball within the orbit above and the oral cavity below. It opens in the lateral nasal wall through the middle meatus, and its floor is separated from the dental roots by a thin plate of bone, so vulnerable invasion by pathogenic organisms through the nose and/or mouth is not rare. Sinusitis of dental origin accounts approximately 10% to 12% of all types of maxillary sinusitis [1]. Odontogenic maxillary sinusitis (OMS) has a special consideration because of differences in pathophysiology, microbiology, and management as compared with non-odontogenic sinusitis. Any disease arising from dental or dentoalveolar structures could violate the floor of the maxillary sinus and may cause OMS [2]. Management of OMS often requires treatment of sinusitis as well its odontogenic source.

Anatomy

The maxillary sinus is one of a series of paranasal sinuses, which includes the ethmoid, sphenoid and frontal sinuses. The maxillary sinus is the first of these paranasal sinuses to develop in the third month of fetal life. Full development of the maxillary sinus is usually reached by the age of 12 to 14 years of age, it corresponds with the eruption of permanent teeth and growth of the alveolar process of the upper jaw [3].

In children and young teenagers, there is considerable distance between the floor of the sinus and the apices of the maxillary teeth, because the sinus has not reached an adult size. The maxillary sinus is bounded by the orbital floor superiorly, the lateral nasal wall medially, lateral wall of the maxilla anteriorly and the dentoalveolar portion of the maxilla inferiorly. The average volume of the maxillary sinus varies between 15 and 20 mL [4]. The roots of the maxillary second molars are in closest proximity to the sinus floor, followed in frequency by the roots of the first molar, third molar, second premolar, and first premolar [5]. However, the floor of the maxillary sinus is consisted of thick cortical bone, not allowing for an easy direct penetration of odontogenic infections into the maxilla sinus. However, the alveolar bone of the maxilla can become thinner with increasing age, leaving a layer of mucoperiosteum with respiratory epithelium between the maxillary sinus and the oral cavity [6, 7]. Also, progressive pneumatization of the sinus which is accompanied with eruption of the permanent teeth may sometimes lead to protrusion of the dental roots into the floor of the sinus [7].

Microbiology

The usual maxillary sinusitis that may follow upper respiratory tract infection is caused mainly by one or more of the following organisms: Streptococcus pneumoniae, Haemophilus influenzae, and Moraxella catarrhalis [8]. However, OMS is completely different in its causal pathogens, the oral bacterial flora which are responsible for odontogenic infections are the same as those implicated in odontogenic maxillary sinusitis. It is usually caused by mixed aerobic and anaerobic organisms including Streptococci spp, Bacteriodes, Viellonella, Corynebacterium, Fusobacterium, and Eikenella [9].

Etiology

The most common etiology of OMS is dentoalveolar surgery or odontogenic infection with violation of the Schneiderian membrane [10]. A recent systematic review studying the causes of OMS from January 1980 to January 2013, among 674 patients, showed that iatrogenic etiology accounted for 65.7% of cases, apical periodontal pathologies for 25.1% and marginal periodontitis for 8.3%. Iatrogenic causes included impacted teeth with dental caries, artificial implants, dental amalgams and oroantral fistula (OAF). In the same study, the most affected maxillary teeth were, in order of frequency: the first molar (35.6%), second molar (22%), third molar (17.4%), and second premolar (14.4%) [11]. In a more recent systematic review, Akhlaghi et al., [12] demonstrated that OAF, as a complication of tooth extraction, was the most common cause of OMS among all dental etiologies.

Pathophysiology

Dental caries and periodontal infections are responsible for most OMS. Dental decay first affects the outermost enamel layer and, if not treated, extends into the inner most dental pulp after dissolution of the middle dentin layer. Once the infection enters the dental pulp, it causes necrosis and formation of pus.

Bacterial toxins and enzymes such as collagenase are considered potent virulence factors in the pathogenesis of bone invasion. The body is unable to eliminate the source of dental infection because the necrotic pulp is protected within the tooth roots. Bacterial toxins and lysosomal enzymes released from phagocytic neutrophils cause tissue damage and bone resorption [13].

Although odontogenic infections are extremely common, the incidence of OMS is not likewise, because the floor of the nose and sinus which is formed of the alveolus is composed of dense cortical bone when compared with the lateral wall of the maxilla [2, 13]. Most odontogenic infections start as soft tissue vestibular or fascial space infections rather than sinusitis as the weak lateral maxillary wall can be affected easily than the floor of the sinus, however, odontogenic infections can drain into the sinus, especially when the roots are in close proximity to the maxillary sinus floor [13].

Some common causes of maxillary sinusitis related to dentistry are the iatrogenic displacement of a maxillary tooth root tip into the sinus during extraction, perforation of the sinus membrane during exodontia, and extrusion of materials used in root canal therapy into the sinus [14]. Also, extraction of posterior maxillary teeth may be complicated with oroantral fistula (OAF) as dental infection may cause thinning out of the maxillary sinus floor. An OAF is a pathologic condition in which the oral and maxillary sinus cavities have a permanent communication by a fibrous channel lined with epithelium. This channel is eventually representing a direct pathway for pathognomonic organisms [15].

Clinical Presentation

Diagnosis of OMS requires a thorough evaluation of the patient's symptoms and past medical and surgical history and their correlation with physical findings.

Symptoms
The main symptoms related to OMS -which is usually unilateral- are:

- Facial pain and/or pressure, especially over the cheek.
- Purulent nasal discharge, usually copious and offensive (due to anaerobic bacteria).
- Nasal congestion, stuffiness and/or obstruction.

- -Cacosmia, due to the offensive odour of discharge.
- Postnasal drip, which may cause throat irritation.
- Toothache, headache, and sometimes earache (caused by referred pain through the trigeminal nerve).
- Nasal regurgitation of fluid, if the condition was associated with oroantral fistula.
- The patient may give a history of recent dental problem or dental extraction.

Dental symptoms can range from acute sharp pain due to an exposed tooth nerve to dull aching pain of dental infection (periapical periodontitis).

However, these symptoms may be difficult to differentiate from other causes of sinusitis. Also, some patients may suffer from sinusitis-like symptoms, such as toothache and nasal congestion, or who presents with minimal sinusitis symptoms and toothache, because the osteomeatal complex is not obstructed and allows drainage and relief of pressure symptoms [15-20].

Clinical Examination

- Inspection of the maxillary teeth, gingiva, buccal mucosa and vestibule for swelling or erythema.
- Palpation of the anterior maxilla may induce tenderness.
- Percussion of the maxillary teeth should be cautiously performed with a dental mirror to see if the pain can be localized to one tooth or if multiple teeth are affected.
- Electric or thermal pulp testing can be used to assess vitality of teeth to further aid in diagnosis.
- Anterior rhinoscopy and diagnostic nasal endoscopy: usually show congested middle meatus with purulent discharge that reforms within seconds after suction.

Oroantral fistula (OAF) can be diagnosed clinically by the Valsalva maneuver or by examining the extraction region with a blunt probe. The presence of OAF may show altering of the voice due to air leakage from the nose or nasal regurgitation of fluid. Additionally, a small amount of purulent discharge may drip through the OAF [15, 13, 21].

Diagnostic Imaging

Radiographic imaging is an essential tool for the diagnosis and management of OMS.

Panoramic radiograph is a standard imaging technique used in dental offices. This view is useful for evaluating the relationship of the maxillary teeth to the sinus, pneumatization, and pseudocysts. It is also used for identifying displaced roots, teeth, or foreign bodies in the sinus.

It has been reported that dental radiographs may miss between 55% and 86% of dental pathology that are involved in OMS [22, 23], so the computed tomography (CT) is considered the gold standard for adequate maxillary sinus imaging because of its high resolution and ability to visualize bone and soft tissue and detect sino-nasal inflammation. Axial and coronal sinus CT views can show the relationship of a periapical abscess with sinus floor defect and can determine the exact location of a foreign body within the maxillary sinus [24-26].

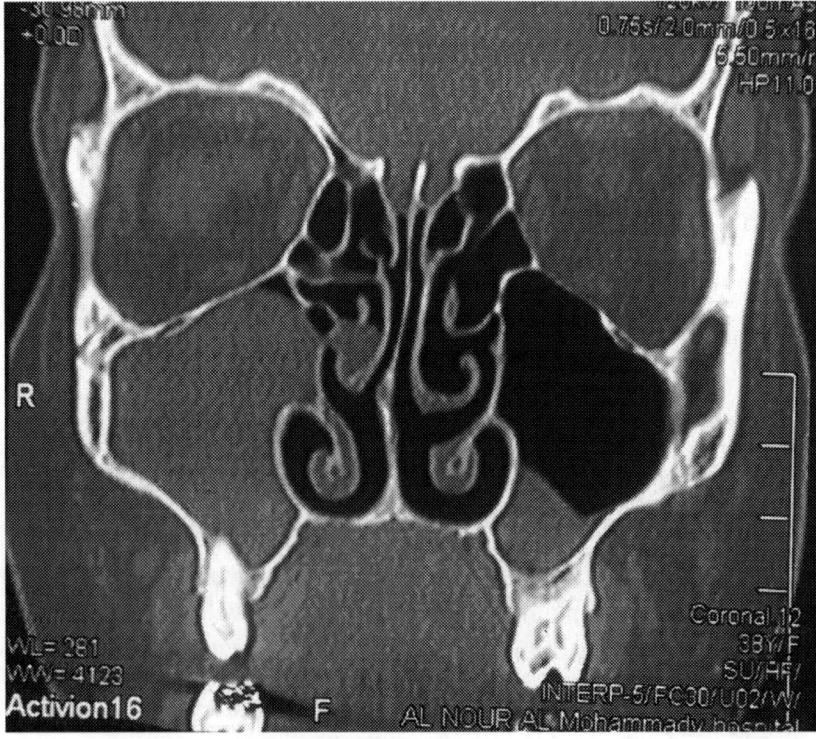

Figure 1. Coronal CT showing total opacity of the right maxillary sinus with the dental root impeded in the floor of the sinus.

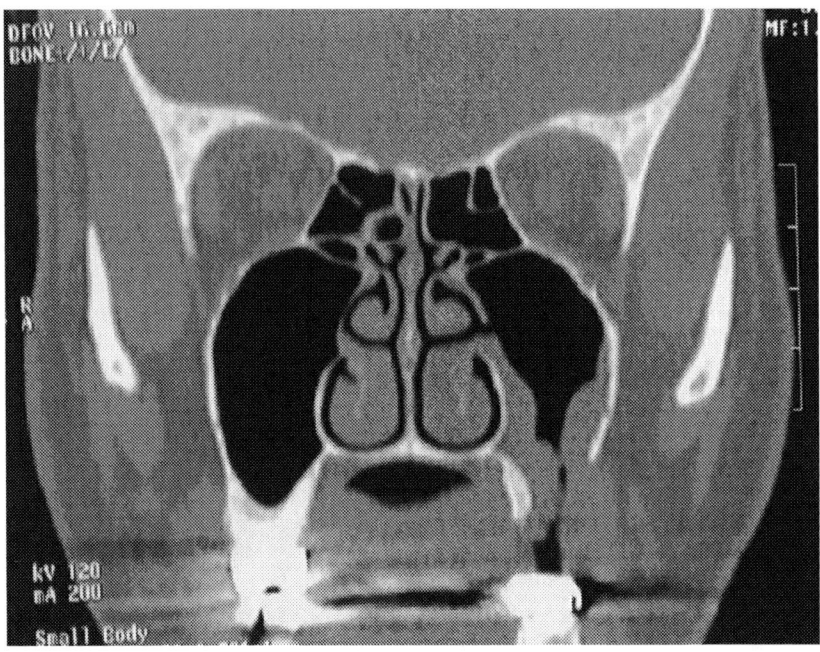

Figure 2. Coronal CT showing oroantral fistula after tooth extraction with mucosal thickening of the left maxillary sinus.

It has been reported that most unilateral isolated maxillary sinusitis cases (more than 70%) are of odontogenic origin [27-29]. OMS is identified on CT images (axial, and coronal planes) as mucosal thickening ≥ 2mm of the maxillary sinus or opacity (Figure 1), associated with a dental focus responsible for sinus pathology, such as OAF (Figure 2), foreign bodies (dental fillings, teeth roots) (Figure 3), periapical abscess, granulomas, or extraction site [30-33].

New advances in 3D imaging systems have introduced cone beam computed tomography (CBCT). The CBCT consumes about 10% of the radiation dose of conventional CT, focusing on bony details. The CBCT is preferred in the field of implant dentistry, in order to assess the thickness of the floor of the maxillary sinus before implantation [17].

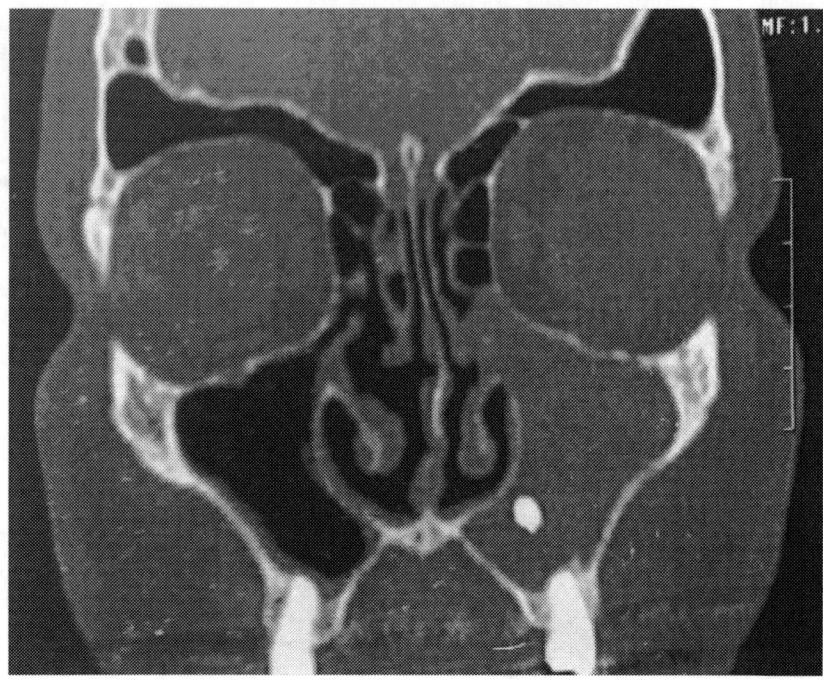

Figure 3. Coronal CT showing total opacification of the left maxillary sinus, with obliteration of the osteomeatal complex and metallic density in the sinus, from previous dental filling extending upwards, causing odontogenic maxillary sinusitis.

Management

Treatment of OMS usually requires combined medical and surgical management with elimination of the source of infection such as: removal of a foreign tooth root from the sinus or treatment of an infected tooth by extraction or root canal therapy [13].

Medical management includes oral antibiotics with adequate sinus and oral flora coverage for one to two weeks. The antibiotic of choice is amoxicillin combined with clavulanate. If the patient has penicillin sensitivity, we can use fluoroquinolones such as moxifloxacin [18, 19, 34]. Macrolide therapy such as Clarithromycin is recommended as one of the medications for treatment of OMS [35]. Systemic and local nasal decongestants with saline nasal irrigation can help greatly in treatment [13]. Also, discontinuation of smoking and avoidance of pollution is very necessary for treatment [15].

Surgical management includes both dental surgery and endoscopic sinus surgery (ESS) [36, 37]. Dental infection source should be treated first through root canal therapy or dental extraction if root canal therapy is unsuccessful [34, 20, 6]. Extraction of maxillary posterior teeth must be done carefully to avoid displacement of root tips into the maxillary sinus or occurrence of OAF [21].

If symptoms persist after management of dental problem, ESS is recommended to drain the sinus, especially if the osteomeatal complex is blocked, and the height of the thickened mucosa is more than one-half of the maxillary sinus [38, 39]. The classical Caldwell-Luc remains an oroantral procedure but has a higher rate of complications; either early complications as: bleeding, facial swelling and infraorbital nerve damage, or long-term complications as: OAF, teeth devitalization and facial paresthesia [21].

Many reports recommend concomitant management of sinus and dental problems to ensure complete resolution of the infection and preventing recurrence [28, 40, 41].

The management of OAF depends on the size of defect, time of diagnosis and presence of OMS [42]. OAF of a duration of more than 3 weeks should be surgically closed, and ESS is required to eliminate granulation tissue and to keep osteomeatal complex patent [43]. If OAF is smaller than 3mm and without epithelization, it often closes spontaneously in the absence of infection [42, 43]. When OAF is larger than 3mm, surgical closure is indicated with buccal advancement flaps. For large bony defects, palatal flaps are recommended [44]. When the soft tissue flaps fail or in case of presence of chronic OAF, autogenous bone grafts derived from chin, retromolar area or iliac crest can be used [42].

Conclusion

Dental causes of maxillary sinusitis are underestimated and may be overlooked by the otolaryngologists, so proper diagnosis is of paramount importance for treatment, as the pathophysiology, microbiology, and treatment differ from those of other types of sinusitis. Sometimes treatment of dental pathology alone is adequate to resolve the condition, however surgical intervention by endoscopic sinus surgery or even Caldwell-Luc operation may be required after treatment of dental problem.

Acknowledgments

Not applicable.

Funding

Self-funded. There are no financial disclosures.

Conflict of Interest

There are no conflicts of interest.

References

[1] Maloney P L, Doku H C. Maxillary sinusitis of odontogenic origin. *J. Can. Dent. Assoc.* 1968; 34(11):591–603. https://pubmed.ncbi.nlm.nih.gov/5247119/.
[2] Abdel-Aziz M, El-Hoshy H, Azooz K, Naguib N, Hussein A. Maxillary sinus mucocele: predisposing factors, clinical presentations, and treatment. *Oral Maxillofac. Surg.* 2017; 21:55–58. https://doi.org/10.1007/s10006-016-0599-5.
[3] Abubaker A O. Applied anatomy of the maxillary sinus. *Oral & Maxillofacial Surgery Clinics.* 1999;11(1):1–13. https://doi.org/10.1016/S1042-3699(20)30280-6.
[4] Sicher H. Oral anatomy. St Louis (MO): C. V. Mosby. Michigan, USA. 4th ed, 1965.
[5] Psillas G, Papaioannou D, Petsali S, Dimas G G, Constantinidis J. Odontogenic maxillary sinusitis: a comprehensive review. *J. Dent. Sci.* 2021;16(1):474-481. https://doi.org/10.1016/j.jds.2020.08.001.
[6] Ferguson M. Rhinosinusitis in oral medicine and dentistry. *Aust. Dent. J.* 2014; 59(3):289-295. https://doi.org/10.1111/adj.12193.
[7] Hauman C H J, Chandler N P, Tong D C. Endodontic implications of the maxillary sinus: a review. *Int. Endod. J.* 2002;35(2):127-141. https://doi.org/10.1046/j.0143-2885.2001.00524.x.
[8] Su W Y, Liu C, Hung S Y, W F Tsai. Bacteriological study in chronic maxillary sinusitis. *Laryngoscope* 1983;93(7):931-934. https://doi.org/10.1288/00005537-198307000-00016.
[9] Sandler N A, Johns F R, Braun T W. Advances in the management of acute and chronic sinusitis. *J. Oral. Maxillofac. Surg.* 1996;54(8):1005-1013. https://doi.org/10.1016/s0278-2391(96)90401-2.
[10] Gaudin R A, Hoehle L P, Smeets R, Heiland M, Caradonna D S, Gray S T & Sedaghat A R.. Impact of odontogenic chronic rhinosinusitis on general health-

related quality of life. *Eur. Arch. Otorhinolaryngol.* 2018;275(6):1477-1482. https://doi.org/10.1007/s00405-018-4977-5.

[11] Lechien J R, Filleul O, de Araujo P C, Hsieh J W, Chantrain G, Saussez S. Chronic maxillary rhinosinusitis of dental origin: a systematic review of 674 patient cases. *Int. J. Otolaryngol.* 2014;2014:465173. https://doi.org/10.1155/2014/465173.

[12] Akhlaghi F, Esmaeelinejad M, Safai P. Etiologies and treatments of odontogenic maxillary sinusitis: a systematic review. *Iran. Red Crescent Med. J.* 2015;17(12): e25536. https://doi.org/10.5812/ircmj.25536.

[13] Mehra P, Murad H. Maxillary sinus disease of odontogenic origin. *Otolaryngol. Clin. North Am.* 2004;37(2):347-364. https://doi.org/10.1016/s0030-6665(03)00171-3.

[14] Timmenga N M, Raghoebar G M, Boering G, van Weissenbruch R. Maxillary sinus function after sinus lifts for the insertion of dental implants. *J. Oral Maxillofac. Surg.* 1997;55(9):936-939. https://doi.org/10.1016/s0278-2391(97)90063-x.

[15] Abdel-Aziz M, Fawaz M, Kamel M, Kamel A, Aljeraisi T. Closure of oroantral fistula with buccal fat pad flap and endoscopic drainage of the maxillary sinus. *J. Craniofac. Surg.* 2018;29: 2153–2155. https://doi.org/10.1097/scs.0000000000004709.

[16] Brook I. Sinusitis of odontogenic origin. *Otolaryngol. Head Neck Surg.* 2006;135 (3):349-355. https://doi.org/10.1016/j.otohns.2005.10.059.

[17] Patel N A, Ferguson B J. Odontogenic sinusitis: an ancient but under-appreciated cause of maxillary sinusitis. *Curr. Opin. Otolaryngol. Head Neck Surg.* 2012; 20(1):24-28. https://doi.org/10.1097/moo.0b013e32834e62ed.

[18] Zirk M, Dreiseidler T, Pohl M, Rothamel D, Buller J, Peters F, Zöller J E & Kreppel M. Odontogenic sinusitis maxillaris: a retrospective study of 121 cases with surgical intervention. *J. Craniomaxillofac. Surg.* 2017;45(4):520-525. https://doi.org/10.1016/j.jcms.2017.01.023.

[19] Vidal F, Coutinho T M, Ferreira D C, de Souza R C, Gonçalves L S. Odontogenic sinusitis: a comprehensive review. *Acta Odontol. Scand.* 2017;75(8):623-633. https://doi.org/10.1080/00016357.2017.1372803.

[20] Little R E, Long C M, Loehrl T A, Poetker D M. Odontogenic sinusitis: a review of the current literature. *Laryngoscope Investig. Otolaryngol.* 2018;3(2):110-114. https://doi.org/10.1002/lio2.147.

[21] Simuntis R, Kubilius R, Vaitkus S. Odontogenic maxillary sinusitis: a review. *Stomatologija* 2014;16(2):39-43. https://pubmed.ncbi.nlm.nih.gov/25209225/.

[22] Longhini A B, Ferguson B J. Clinical aspects of odontogenic maxillary sinusitis: a case series. *Int. Forum Allergy Rhinol.* 2011;1(5):409-415. https://doi.org/10.1002/alr.20058.

[23] Melén I, Lindahl L, Andréasson L, Rundcrantz H. Chronic maxillary sinusitis. Definition, diagnosis and relation to dental infections and nasal polyposis. *Acta Otolaryngol.* 1986;101(3-4):320-327. https://doi.org/10.3109/00016488609132845.

[24] Lofthag-Hansen S, Huumonen S, Gröndahl K, Gröndahl H. Limited cone-beam CT and intraoral radiography for the diagnosisof periapical pathology. *Oral Surg. Oral Med. Oral Pathol. Oral Radiol. Endod.* 2007;103(1):114-119. https://doi.org/10.1016/j.tripleo.2006.01.001.

[25] Guijarro-Martínez R, Swennen G R J. Cone-beam computerized tomography imaging and analysis of the upper airway: a systematic review of the literature. *Int. J. Oral Maxillofac. Surg.* 2011;40(11):1227-1237. https://doi.org/10.1016/j.ijom.2011.06.017.

[26] Misch K A, Yi E S, Sarment D P. Accuracy of cone beam computed tomography for periodontal defect measurements. *J. Periodontol.* 2006;77(7):1261-1266. https://doi.org/10.1902/jop.2006.050367.

[27] Troeltzsch M, Pache C, Troeltzsch M, Kaeppler G, Ehrenfeld M, Otto S & Probst F. Etiology and clinical characteristics of symptomatic unilateral maxillary sinusitis: a review of 174 cases. *J. Craniomaxillofac. Surg.* 2015;43(8):1522-1529. https://doi.org/10.1016/j.jcms.2015.07.021.

[28] Lee K C, Lee S J. Clinical features and treatments of odontogenic sinusitis. *Yonsei Med. J.* 2010;51(6):932-937. https://doi.org/10.3349/ymj.2010.51.6.932.

[29] Matsumoto Y, Ikeda T, Yokoi H, Kohno N. Association between odontogenic infections and unilateral sinus opacification. *Auris Nasus Larynx.* 2015;42(4):288-293. https://doi.org/10.1016/j.anl.2014.12.006.

[30] Capelli M, Gatti P. Radiological study of maxillary sinus using CBCT: relationship between mucosal thickening and common anatomic variants in chronic rhinosinusitis. *J. Clin. Diagn. Res.* 2016;10(11):MC07-MC10. https://doi.org/10.7860/jcdr/2016/22365.8931.

[31] Pokorny A, Tataryn R. Clinical and radiologic findings in a case series of maxillary sinusitis of dental origin. *Int. Forum Allergy Rhinol.* 2013;3(12):973-979. https://doi.org/10.1002/alr.21212.

[32] Maska B, Lin G, Othman A, Behdin S, Travan S, Benavides E & Kapila Y. Dental implants and grafting success remain high despite large variations in maxillary sinus mucosal thickening. *Int. J. Implant Dent.* 2017;3(1):1. https://doi.org/10.1186/s40729-017-0064-8.

[33] Guerra-Pereira I, Vaz P, Faria-Almeida R, Braga A, Felino A. CT maxillary sinus evaluation--A retrospective cohort study. *Med. Oral Patol. Oral Cir. Bucal* 2015;20(4):e419-426. https://doi.org/10.4317/medoral.20513.

[34] Workman A D, Granquist E J, Adappa N D. Odontogenic sinusitis: developments in diagnosis, microbiology, and treatment. *Curr. Opin. Otolaryngol. Head Neck Surg.* 2018;26(1):27-33. https://doi.org/10.1097/moo.0000000000000430.

[35] Shimizu, T.; Suzaki, H. Past, present and future of macrolide therapy for chronic rhinosinusitis in Japan. *Auris Nasus Larynx* 2016;43(2):131-136. https://doi.org/10.1016/j.anl.2015.08.014.

[36] Wang K L, Nichols B G, Poetker D M, Loehrl T A. Odontogenic sinusitis: a case studying diagnosis and management. *Int. Forum Allergy Rhinol.* 2015;5(7):597-601. https://doi.org/10.1002/alr.21504.

[37] Aukštakalnis R, Simonavičiūtė R, Simuntis R. Treatment options for odontogenic maxillary sinusitis: a review. *Stomatologija* 2018;20(1):22-26. https://pubmed.ncbi.nlm.nih.gov/29806655/.

[38] Mattos J L, Ferguson B J, Lee S. Predictive factors in patients undergoing endoscopic sinus surgery for odontogenic sinusitis. *Int. Forum Allergy Rhinol.* 2016;6(7):697-700. https://doi.org/10.1002/alr.21736.

[39] Chen Y, Huang C, Chang P, Chen C, Wu C, Fu C & Lee T. The characteristics and new treatment paradigm of dental implant-related chronic rhinosinusitis. *Am. J. Rhinol. Allergy* 2013;27(3):237-244. https://doi.org/10.2500/ajra.2013.27.3884.

[40] Felisati G, Chiapasco M, Lozza P, Saibene A M, Pipolo C, Zaniboni M, Biglioli F & Borloni R. Sinonasal complications resulting from dental treatment: outcome-oriented proposal of classification and surgical protocol. *Am. J. Rhinol. Allergy* 2013;27(4): e101-106. https://doi.org/10.2500/ajra.2013.27.3936.

[41] Saibene A M, Collurà F, Pipolo C, Bulfamante A M, Lozza P, Maccari A, Arnone F, Ghelma F, Allevi F, Biglioli F, Chiapasco M, Portaleone S M, Scotti A, Borloni R & Felisati G. Odontogenic rhinosinusitis and sinonasal complications of dental disease or treatment: prospective validation of a classification and treatment protocol. *Eur. Arch. Otorhinolaryngol.* 2019;276(2):401-406. https://doi.org/10.1007/s00405-018-5220-0.

[42] Krishanappa S K K, Prashanti E, Sumanth K N, Naresh S, Moe S, Aggarwal H & Mathew R J. Interventions for treating oro-antral communications and fistulae due to dental procedures. *Cochrane Database Syst. Rev.* 2018;8:CD011784. https://doi.org/10.1002/14651858.cd011784.pub2.

[43] Borgonovo A E, Berardinelli F V, Favale M, Maiorana C. Surgical options in oroantral fistula treatment. *Open Dent. J.* 2012;6:94-98. https://doi.org/10.2174/1874210601206010094.

[44] Yalçın S, Oncü B, Emes Y, Atalay B, Aktaş I. Surgical treatment of oroantral fistulas: a clinical study of 23 cases. *J. Oral Maxillofac. Surg.* 2011;69(2):333-339. https://doi.org/10.1016/j.joms.2010.02.061.

Index

A

agenesis, 1, 7, 8, 9
anatomy, 41, 47, 55, 60, 61, 63, 64, 65, 66, 72, 75, 76, 77, 80, 81, 82, 91, 94, 102
antrostomy, 32, 41, 85, 90, 91
auto immune disease, 1, 26, 27, 28

B

bacterial infections, 15, 48, 51
biopsy, 1, 3, 12, 17, 19, 22, 40, 41

C

cholesteatoma, 39, 40, 41, 44
classification, 21, 80, 85, 86, 89, 91, 105
CT scan, 1, 2, 4, 6, 7, 8, 9, 10, 11, 12, 13, 15, 17, 18, 19, 22, 26, 29, 31, 33, 36, 38, 40, 81, 85, 86, 88, 89, 90

D

dental infection, v, vii, 46, 54, 58, 63, 64, 65, 68, 69, 70, 72, 74, 75, 76, 93, 96, 97, 103
dental infections oral hygiene, 46
dental pathology, 64, 69, 93, 98, 101

E

embryology, 80, 82, 91
endoscopic surgery, 23, 32, 87
endoscopy, 1, 2, 3, 8, 10, 12, 17, 18, 28, 40, 41, 43, 87, 97
ethmoid, 44, 80, 82, 83, 84, 88, 89, 92, 94

F

foreign body maxillary sinus, 1
fungal infections, 50, 52

H

hypoplasia, 8, 9, 35, 79, 80, 84, 85, 86, 91, 92

I

inflammatory myofibroblastic tumor (IMT), 21, 22, 23, 24, 42
infundibulum, 82, 83, 86, 88, 89

L

leprosy, 14, 16, 17, 25, 42

M

maxillary sinus (MS), v, vii, 1, 2, 3, 4, 5, 6, 7, 8, 9, 10, 11, 12, 14, 15, 16, 18, 19, 20, 21, 22, 24, 25, 26, 28, 29, 31, 32, 33, 34, 35, 36, 37, 38, 39, 40, 41, 42, 43, 44, 45, 46, 47, 48, 49, 50, 51, 52, 53, 54, 55, 56, 57, 58, 59, 60, 61, 62, 63, 64, 65, 66, 67, 68, 69, 70, 71, 72, 73, 74, 75, 76, 77, 79, 80, 81, 82, 83, 84, 85, 86, 87, 88, 89, 90, 91, 93, 94, 95, 96, 98, 99, 100, 101, 102, 103, 104
maxillary sinus hypoplasia (MSH), v, vii, 35, 79, 80, 81, 84, 85, 86, 90, 91
maxillary sinus tumor, 18, 39
maxillary sinusitis, v, vii, 45, 46, 47, 48, 49, 50, 51, 52, 53, 54, 55, 56, 57, 58, 59, 60, 61, 62, 63, 64, 76, 77, 81, 93, 94, 95, 96, 99, 100, 101, 102, 103, 104

microbiology, 45, 46, 47, 53, 56, 59, 60, 61, 62, 93, 94, 95, 101, 104
middle meatotomy, 1, 2, 19, 37
MRI indicate size, 22
multidisciplinary care, v, vii, 45, 46, 59

N

nose, 9, 25, 42, 43, 44, 81, 83, 94, 96, 97

O

odontogenic infection, 12, 49, 54, 64, 94, 95, 96, 104
odontogenic origin, 46, 47, 52, 53, 54, 56, 60, 61, 76, 77, 99, 102, 103
odontogenic sinusitis, 52, 53, 54, 56, 60, 61, 93, 94, 104
orbit, 18, 29, 35, 36, 66, 79, 80, 82, 88, 89, 94
oroantral fistula, 33, 93, 95, 96, 97, 99, 103, 105

P

positron emission tomography-computed tomography (PET CT), 22

S

semiology, 18

silent sinus syndrome (SSS), 34, 35, 36, 37, 43, 88, 89, 92
sinus, vii, 1, 2, 3, 4, 5, 6, 7, 8, 9, 11, 12, 14, 17, 18, 19, 20, 22, 25, 26, 28, 29, 31, 32, 34, 35, 36, 37, 38, 39, 40, 41, 42, 45, 46, 47, 49, 50, 51, 52, 53, 54, 55, 56, 57, 58, 59, 60, 61, 63, 64, 65, 66, 67, 68, 69, 70, 71, 72, 74, 75, 76, 79, 80, 81, 82, 83, 84, 85, 86, 87, 88, 89, 90, 91, 92, 93, 94, 96, 98, 99, 100, 101, 102, 103, 104
sinus endoscopy, 1
sinusitis, vii, 8, 10, 13, 25, 32, 33, 42, 43, 45, 46, 47, 48, 49, 50, 51, 52, 53, 54, 55, 56, 57, 59, 60, 61, 63, 64, 74, 76, 77, 80, 84, 85, 86, 89, 91, 93, 94, 95, 96, 97, 101, 102, 103, 104

T

trigeminal nerve, 3, 67, 97

U

uncinate process, 35, 36, 82, 83, 84, 85, 86, 91

V

viral Infections, 50, 52
viruses, 48, 50, 51, 52, 55, 60